Basic Guide to Dental Radiography

BASIC GUIDE TO DENTAL RADIOGRAPHY

Tim Reynolds
Education Consultant in Dental Radiology

WILEY Blackwell

This edition first published 2016
© 2016 by John Wiley & Sons, Ltd

Registered Office
John Wiley & Sons, Ltd, The Atrium, Southern Gate, Chichester, West Sussex, PO19 8SQ, UK

Editorial Offices
9600 Garsington Road, Oxford, OX4 2DQ, UK
The Atrium, Southern Gate, Chichester, West Sussex, PO19 8SQ, UK
1606 Golden Aspen Drive, Suites 103 and 104, Ames, Iowa 50010, USA

For details of our global editorial offices, for customer services and for information about how to apply for permission to reuse the copyright material in this book please see our website at www.wiley.com/wiley-blackwell.

Library of Congress Cataloging-in-Publication Data

Names: Reynolds, Tim (Lecturer in radiography), author.
Title: Basic guide to dental radiography / Tim Reynolds.
Description: Chichester, West Sussex ; Ames, Iowa : John Wiley & Sons Ltd., 2016. |
  Includes bibliographical references and index.
Identifiers: LCCN 2016024804 | ISBN 9780470673126 (pbk.) | ISBN 9781118916261 (Adobe PDF) |
  ISBN 9781118916278 (epub)
Subjects: MESH: Radiography, Dental–methods
Classification: LCC RK309 | NLM WN 230 | DDC 617.6/07572–dc23
  LC record available at https://lccn.loc.gov/2016024804

A catalogue record for this book is available from the British Library.

Wiley also publishes its books in a variety of electronic formats. Some content that appears in print may not be available in electronic books.

Cover image: ©gmutlu/gettyimages

1   2016

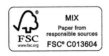

I dedicate this text to R. F. Farr, Chacket, John Ball, Brian Murphy and to my father who passed away on 27 September 2013 and will never see this text published though he asked me about it often during its preparation.

Contents

Acknowledgements

A massive thank you is due to my wife and two young children for putting up with the hours I have spent, effectively, an absent husband and father while putting together this text.

They have missed me and put up with it in good grace; the advantage of being able to quietly get on with the work has been a blessing although there were times that I would have welcomed an interruption.

Also many additional thanks to my wife for allowing me to take and to publish a number of photographs of her in less than flattering circumstances (film holders in position).

From my past I must thank Mr R. F. Farr and Dr Chacket, both formerly of the Queen Elizabeth Hospital Birmingham.

Also Mr John Ball, sadly no longer with us; he was formerly Deputy Principal of the Dudley Road School of Radiography.

The three of them together must form what is probably the greatest physics teaching team ever. Whatever understanding I have of the physics, geometry and theories of imaging in radiography comes largely from their teaching.

Lastly, Mr Brian Murphy, formerly Principal of the Dudley Road School of Radiography; he was possessed of the greatest breadth of knowledge of radiography that I have ever encountered.

Like John Ball, Brian is no longer with us but will always be remembered; he was a great teacher, mentor and in later years a very good friend. The career that I built was through his example and his guidance; I owe him much and he will not be forgotten.

These four together have provided the vast bulk of the information contained within these pages.

Chapter 1

General physics

ATOMS AND MOLECULES

Whenever setting out on a project of this type, it is difficult to know what to use as your starting point.

Let us start by looking at what makes up the world as we know it.

We look around and see lakes, mountains, fields, etc., but what if we could look into these things and see what makes them what they are?

We would see atoms and molecules.

There can't be many people who have not heard of these, but what are they?

Atoms and molecules are linked to elements and compounds (here is the problem – almost every time we mention anything, it will lead us straight to something else we need to know).

Elements are single chemical substances such as oxygen, hydrogen, sulphur, etc. We can take a large amount of an element and keep cutting it down to make it smaller and smaller, but there is a limit to how small we can make it.

We come to a point where all that we have is a single atom of the substance; if we then cut it to an even smaller size, we will be breaking down the atom, and it will no longer be that particular substance.

> • Atoms are the smallest particle of an element that can exist and still behave as that element.

Breaking down an atom eventually produces just a collection of the bits that make up the atom.

Here we go again! What is smaller than an atom? Or what are atoms made of?

There are many so-called fundamental particles that make up the atoms that provide the basic building blocks for all of the things that we see, touch and know of. Some of these fundamental particles are only now being discovered.

For the purposes of fulfilling the basic guide brief, we will concentrate on only three types of particle: protons, neutrons and electrons.

Basic Guide to Dental Radiography, First Edition. Tim Reynolds.
© 2016 John Wiley & Sons, Ltd. Published 2016 by John Wiley & Sons, Ltd.

Protons and neutrons are large (that's relative; remember we would need very powerful microscope to see even these particles), and electrons are small.

To represent the difference in these particles in a way you can visualise, think of placing a single grape pip on the ground and then standing a person 6 ft tall next to it.

The grape pip represents the size of an electron, and the 6-ft-tall person the size of a proton or a neutron. Protons and neutrons are slightly different in size, but for our purposes they can be considered to be the same, but electrons are 1840 times smaller than either of the other two particles.

The protons and electrons each have an electrical charge and these charges are of opposite poles (like the two ends of a battery). The protons have a positive charge (+ve), and the electrons a negative charge (−ve).

Despite the relative size difference of the particles, the two charges, although opposite poles (or signs), are of equal size or strength.

So the positive charge on one large proton is completely cancelled out by the negative charge on one tiny electron.

Neutrons have no charge at all (they are neutral).

How do these particles fit together to make an atom?

Figure 1.1 shows what has become an accepted idea of the appearance of an atom.

There is a large central nucleus, containing protons and neutrons with the electrons circling in a number of orbits at different distances from the nucleus. These orbits have traditionally been called electron shells or energy shells.

This model will be adequate for our understanding, but do remember that the electron orbits are not all in the same plane. The atom is three-dimensional, and the electron orbits taken all together would make a pattern much more like looking at a football.

This makes sense if you think of the electron orbits as actual shells; they completely surround the nucleus much like the layers of an onion. This is difficult to demonstrate on a flat page, and we have become used to the picture as shown (Figure 1.1) with lots of circles having the same centre.

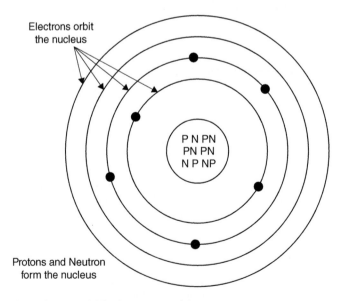

Figure 1.1 Classic basic model for the structure of the atom

The number of protons in the nucleus tells us what sort of atom it is. A nucleus containing 6 protons would be a carbon nucleus, 11 protons sodium, and 82 protons lead. The number of protons present is the atomic number of the element and of course of the atom; the number of protons in fact tells us what chemical substance the atom is.

The protons in the nucleus all have a positive charge, and the tendency for positive charges is to push each other apart just like two magnetic north or two south poles would. They need something to keep them from pushing each other away; this function is performed by the neutrons. The neutrons don't do this job alone, but for the purposes of this particular text, we need look no further into nuclear forces. At very low atomic numbers, there will be equal numbers of protons and neutrons; however as atomic number increases, the higher concentration of positively charged protons needs a higher number of neutrons to overcome the forces of repulsion between them.

The number of electrons in each orbit is specific and is determined by the following formula:

$$E = 2n^2$$

where E is the number of electrons and n is the number of the electron shell.

So, the closest shell to the nucleus is number 1. In that shell, you can have 2×1^2 electrons.

1^2 is 1×1 so that 1 multiplied by 2 tells us we can have two electrons in the first shell. In the second shell we can have 2×2^2. So 2×2 (n^2) = 4 multiplied by 2 gives 8. In the third shell 2×3^2 gives 2×9. So 18 electrons would be allowed in shell 3.

No electrons can be positioned in shell 2 if shell 1 is not full and none in shell 3 if shell 2 is not full. That is to say that all inner shells must be filled before outer shells can contain any electrons. If an electron were removed from an inner shell, then one would move down from an outer shell to fill the gap. (This becomes important when we consider the effects of exposure to radiation.)

The process works like this because atoms always exist in their lowest energy state (ground state) and inner shell electrons are the low energy ones. So if we take out a low-energy inner shell electron, the atom is at a higher level of energy than it could be, so an electron from a shell further out falls to fill the gap and in the process gives up some of its energy.

The electron filling the gap will give up some energy because it can only be in the lower shell if it has the correct level of energy. This process will continue until the exchange takes place at the outermost shell of the atom. There will then be an electron space free in the outer shell of the atom (the one that is the greatest distance from the nucleus) (Figure 1.2).

From the previous descriptions, it is clear that most of the mass of an atom (it's easier to think of this as weight or just the solid material) is in the nucleus of the atom.

A carbon atom with 6 protons and 6 neutrons (there are forms of carbon with a different number of neutrons, but we are not concerned with isotopes in this text) will have 6 electrons circulating in two discrete orbits (2 in shell 1 and 4 in shell 2). So in terms of the sheer bulk of material in relative terms, the electrons account for six times one, and the nucleus for 12 times 1840.

This means the solid matter that makes up an atom is mostly contained in the nucleus (where the big particles are). However if we look at the overall size of the atom (from one side of the outer electron shell to the other), most of it is not made up of material at all but of empty space. Even taking into account the relatively large particles in the nucleus,

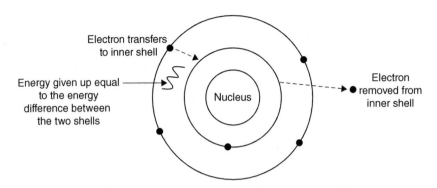

Figure 1.2 Redistribution of electrons to the atoms' lowest energy state

all elements including things like lead have atoms that are almost entirely free space. This is sort of like a large fishing net on a trawler; if the net was 50 yd by 50 yd, the overall size is massive, but if you just put the material making the net together, it would be tiny by comparison; the overall measurements of the net are made up mostly of the gaps between the materials.

To round off our investigation of atoms, the following is presented.

The electron shells are not called 1, 2 and 3 but are denoted by letters, number 1 is K, number 2 L, number 3 M, and so on; this form of atomic structure will be found in any basic science or physics book though not in advanced texts on the topic. The shell numbers simply allow us to calculate the number of electrons allowed to be in the particular orbit or shell.

On page 1 when we started talking about atoms, we also mentioned molecules, so we now need to bring those back into our thinking.

When we introduced molecules we said the atoms and molecules were linked to elements and compounds.

We have discussed elements, so what are compounds?

A compound is a combination of two or more elements; a combination that everyone knows is H_2O (water).

The formula indicates that there are two hydrogen atoms and one of oxygen. The collection of three atoms shown is a molecule of water. If we try to cut this down to make an even smaller amount, we end up with something that is no longer water. Take the oxygen out and we simply have two atoms of hydrogen; if we take away an hydrogen atom, we have an hydroxide or an hydroxyl radical.

- A molecule is the smallest particle of a compound that can exist and still behave chemically as that compound.

NB: Molecules are not always made up of atoms from different elements; a molecule is a collection of two or more atoms; they could be two atoms of oxygen or any other element.

Why do the atoms of different elements join together to make molecules of compounds? We could get into a big discussion on chemistry here, but we don't actually need to.

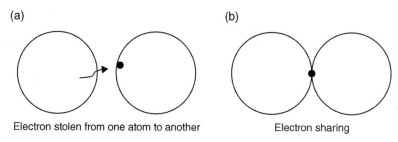

(a)

(b)

Electron stolen from one atom to another

Electron sharing

Figure 1.3 (a) Atomic bonding (ionic bond). (b) Atomic bonding (covalent bond)

The simplest way of thinking about the reason for these combinations is that all atoms would like their outer electron shell to be full.

If it isn't then they may combine with another material by taking an electron from it; the materials are then held together by a tug of war over the electron because both atoms want it in their outer shell. This type of joining is called an ionic bond (Figure 1.3a).

Another way in which atoms join is that they may share electrons, so that electrons in their outer shells effectively take part in the outer orbit of both atoms; this is a bit more like walking hand in hand down the road with your partner. This is a covalent (sharing) bond (Figure 1.3b).

We have just learned that the outer shell electrons of an atom give the atom its chemical properties; they are what make the atoms of one element bond with atoms of other elements to make the molecules of a compound. We can consider outer shell electrons to be 'chemical glue'.

Remember previously we said the electrons could not be put into outer shells if inner ones were not filled and that if an electron were taken out of an inner shell, its place would be taken by an electron from a shell further out; this process continues until all inner shell vacancies are filled. The result is that following the final movement, there will be a vacancy on the electron shell most remote from the nucleus (the outside shell). This shell gives the atom its chemical properties, so removing electrons from atoms changes their chemical properties. This is an important concept for understanding the biological effects of X-rays.

ENERGY

The previous section looked at the material (stuff) that makes up the world that we live in. Next thing to consider is what makes things work.

As always we should look for clues in what we do or say every day. If you have had a tough couple of days, worked hard and not slept, you come to a point where you say I have had it, I can't go on, and I've got no energy.

When we want to measure either amount of energy stored or used in a system, we might use a different word to describe it in different situations. There is however a general measure of energy that can be used in any circumstances; it is the Joule.

If you have ever been on a diet and watching food labels, you will have seen a statement telling you the number of joules (usually kilojoules (kJ)), so you can work out how many chocolate bars you need to just get you through the day.

So there it is, energy is what enables us to do work (or to play); some physics books actually define energy as the ability to do work.

There are lists indicating many sorts of energy, but if you look carefully at each, you can pretty well fit them all into one of the following two categories: kinetic energy (KE) and potential energy (PE).

Kinetic energy is the energy of movement, and potential energy is stored energy.

In classical physics we have the conservation of energy that says energy can be neither created nor destroyed but merely changed from one form to another.

In a very simple example of energy conversion, we could consider lifting a weight from the floor to a shelf six feet high. The work that you have done in lifting that weight is now stored as potential energy. If the weight is then pushed off the shelf, it falls; during the fall it has kinetic energy (energy of movement). On hitting the floor there will be a loud bang (sound energy), and a little heat will be produced.

The potential energy has been through two changes: potential energy to kinetic and kinetic energy to sound and heat.

Other types of energy that you might see are electrical and chemical; there are others but we do not need to produce a full list to examine the basic principles.

What type of energy is electrical energy? The answer is, 'it depends what it's doing'.

Electrical Energy in a battery is potential energy; it's there but it is doing nothing, but it does have the potential to make a small light bulb or a small electric motor work. When we turn on the switch to make the battery work, the electrical energy travels along wires or another form of connection to the item we want to work. As the electrical energy travels to the object, it is kinetic in nature (energy of movement). When the electrical energy arrives at its destination, it may be converted again. In a light bulb, it will produce light and heat energy. In a small electric motor, it will produce mechanical kinetic energy (it makes the motor parts move).

Heat energy is kinetic energy. We think of things as hot or cold, and we can feel the difference what we can't see is happening to the molecules in a hot or cold object.

When objects are cool the molecules do not move very much; as we increase the temperature, they move around more and much more quickly. We can see some evidence of this because we all know that as things warm up, they get bigger (expand). They do this because the molecules are moving about more. You can do an experiment to show this with a group of friends. Get them together and stand as still as you can and as close together. You will be able to fit into quite a small space. Now start moving around as if you might be dancing, and see how much more space is required by the group as a whole. This is exactly what happens when an object is heated (Figure 1.4).

When the bar is cold, the individual molecules (represented by the circles) are packed close together. After heating each molecule will move about; let's say they move backwards and forwards between the lines I have set at each side of them. Look at how much longer the bar would have to be to allow this movement.

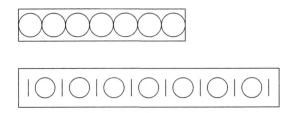

Figure 1.4 Explanation of expansion due to heating

When we give objects heat energy, we change their temperature. Heat energy can be transferred (moved) in three ways: conduction, convection and radiation.

Conduction of heat energy is through simple physical contact. The heat energy is passed from one molecule or one body to another. If you were standing in that closely packed group of friends and you were the only one that wanted to dance, the person next to you would soon be forced to move and then the one next to them and so on. If you were standing next to another group, they would also soon be forced to start moving.

Convection is how heat is generally transferred in liquids and gases; the warm molecules actually move from one area to another. If you have a bath with the tap set at one end and you fill it with cold water and then put hot water in the tap end, you can make the other end warm by swishing the water round with your hand. Eventually all of the water will have the same temperature because hot mixes with cold and the hot water molecules pass some of their heat to the cooler ones through conduction. So there will always be some conduction along with convection simply because the molecules are in contact with each other.

Radiation is the most difficult to understand as it does not pass through particles by movement or contact; in fact it does not pass through particles at all as it can move through a perfect vacuum (i.e. an area containing not even a single fundamental particle). Radiation is how we can feel the heat of the sun as it passes through millions of miles of space and gives kinetic energy to the molecules of our skin.

Large amounts of heat energy are produced when an X-ray machine is working, and we have to be able to move it away to stop it from damaging the machine, so these heat transfer methods are important during the production of X-rays.

ELECTRICAL ENERGY

The basis of electrical energy comes from the existence of the two types of electric charge that we have mentioned already, the positive charge on a proton and the negative charge on an electron. Electric charge is measured by a unit called the coulomb (C). This is a relatively large unit of charge, and for there to be 1 C of negative charge, we would need to collect 6×10^{18} electrons (that's 6 followed by 18 noughts), or the same number of protons will produce 1 C of positive charge.

These charges have an influence on each other; forces will exist between them. If the charges are alike (two positives or two negatives), they will push each other away (Figure 1.5a and 1.5b). If they are unlike charges, they will attract each other (Figure 1.5c). This force is always present, it's strength will depend the size of the charges and a number of other factors.

The force of attraction can also be seen in objects that have no charge if a large enough external charge is brought close to it. This happens because the electron orbits around an atom can be distorted (have their shape changed) (Figure 1.6).

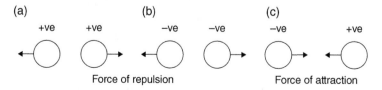

Figure 1.5 (a, b and c) Electric forces

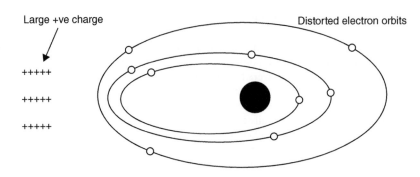

Figure 1.6 Charge induction through electron orbit distortion

The electron orbits have been distorted by the close positive charge; the electrons have been attracted to it, and the orbits have become elliptical. The positive charges of the nucleus are effectively further from the large external positive charge than the electrons are, and the two objects are attracted towards each other because the atom behaves as if it is negatively charged. If the external electric charge had been a negative one, the electrons would have been pushed away, and there would effectively be a force of repulsion between the external charge and the atom.

This effect has been induced by the external charge.

In some materials some of the electrons are free to move so that when a large positive charge is applied, the electrons will move through the material.

Electrical charge then can be the driving force to make other charges move – we call this driving force, voltage. When electrical charges do move, they are called current.

Voltage (it will not surprise you to learn) is measured in volts and current is measured in amps (Amperes).

1 Amp of current flows when 1 Coulomb of charge passes a point in 1 second (that's a lot of electrons, 6×10^{18} moving past a particular point past in 1 second).

When electrical charges move it is almost always electrons that move, simply because they are small enough to be influenced by other charges. In addition to being very large (atomically speaking), protons are usually firmly fixed together with other protons and the other large particle neutrons, right in the middle of the atom in the nucleus.

We have previously looked at the structure of the atom and described a number of electron shells, but rather than shells they become energy bands (it's like comparing a country lane to a six-lane motorway). The shells become bands because of the influence of all the other atoms around them.

We also talked about the outer shell (band) being responsible for the chemical (bonding) properties of the atom – this band is called the valence band. There is however another band outside of this one – it's called the conduction band. As the name implies, this is where electrical conduction (the movement of electrons) takes place.

Of course not all materials conduct electricity; if they did we would not be able to walk around our own homes without getting a shock as we have electrical wires behind all of our walls.

So what makes the difference?

The conduction band of electrons is an area where, effectively, the electrons belong to the atom but are not firmly fixed to the nucleus; they are free to move around as long as

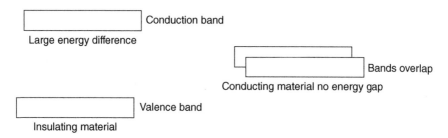

Figure 1.7 Valence and conduction bands in conductors and insulators

there is some influence (e.g. voltage) to cause that movement. The atom doesn't change because for every electron that moves out, one will move in.

The difference between an electrical conductor and an insulator is the energy difference (how big a step) between the valence band and the conduction band. In the valence band the electrons are fixed firmly in place; in the conduction band they are free to move under the influence of an applied voltage.

In an insulating material there is a large energy difference, and electrons are highly unlikely to ever have an energy increase sufficient to take them into the conduction band. In a conducting material the bands actually overlap so that there are always unattached electrons free to move through the material (Figure 1.7).

Even when electrons move there will still be the correct number of electrons associated with each atom because as electrons move out of one atom into the next, they are immediately replaced by electrons from the atom on the other side.

There are also semiconducting materials where the gap is small, and small amounts of energy can make electrons move into the conduction band.

ELECTRIC CURRENT

For current to flow there must be a closed circuit, a complete uninterrupted path for the voltage to be applied across and for the electrons to flow in. When using a light switch or pressing the exposure button on an X-ray machine, we are simply completing the circuit (Figure 1.8).

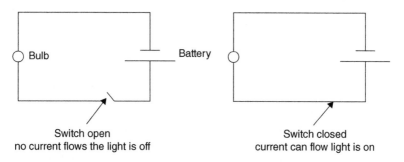

Figure 1.8 Open and closed circuits

GENERAL PHYSICS

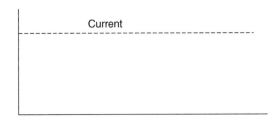

Figure 1.9 Direct current flow

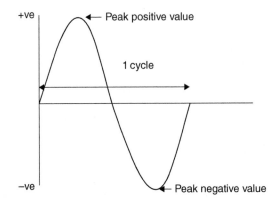

Figure 1.10 Alternating current flow

There are two ways in which electric current can flow in a circuit – there is direct current (DC) and alternating current (AC).

DC does not vary as it is the sort of current flow we get from a battery.

Seen in the form of a graph, DC looks like that shown in Figure 1.9.

With AC the movement effectively shuffles backwards and forwards as the voltage at each end of the connection changes constantly from positive to negative and back again (alternates between positive and negative).

Seen on a graph AC looks like that shown in Figure 1.10.

Both current and voltage follow this positive/negative pattern, but are not exactly the same shape.

The full progress of current and voltage from zero to positive peak down to negative peak and back to zero is called a cycle. Frequency is the number of times a supply goes through a full cycle in a second. The frequency of mains electricity in the United Kingdom is 50 Hz (that's 50 cycles per second).

This shunting backwards and forwards of electrons may seem like a waste of time, but sometimes it is not important for electrons to arrive at a particular point simply that they are moving because the movement of electrons in a conductor has a number of important effects.

Looking at the graph it is clear that as we look at the average value of voltage or current, it will be zero because they both spend exactly the same amount of time being positive and then negative.

The average value of voltage and current being zero makes it seem that no energy is used when passing an AC.

This however is not the case as to move the electrons; work still has to be done against the electrical resistance.

Electrical resistance tells us how easy or difficult it is to move current through a particular material or through a different sample of the same material. Many factors have an effect on the resistance, but discussion of these factors falls outside the scope of this text.

Rather than use average current or voltage to describe the effects within an electrical circuit, we use effective current and effective voltage.

The effective current or voltage in an alternating supply is that Direct Current or voltage which acting for the same period of time would result in the use of the same amount of energy as the alternating supply.

Effective current or voltage is also referred to as the root mean square (RMS) value.

The RMS value of both current and voltage is a little more than 70% (seven tenths) of the maximum peak value. We need to know this when calculating things like power (energy used) in a circuit. You will be pleased to know that this study will not include such calculations.

The knowledge we have so far of atoms, molecules, energy and electricity gives us most of what we need to know about how X-rays are produced for diagnostic purposes.

Chapter 2

X-ray production

The principles of atomic structure, electric potential, current flow and energy conversion are all we need to know in order to understand, at a basic level, the production of the X-ray beam we use to examine our patients.

One thing we need to add to the aforementioned list is an evacuated glass envelope. This is a closed glass tube that has been turned into a perfect vacuum. To produce the perfect vacuum, all the air has been sucked out to the point where not a single particle, proton, neutron or electron remains inside the tube.

The reason we need this perfect vacuum is that we need to accelerate electrons across the tube (we will call these electrons filament electrons) at very high speed. That is, we will give them lots of kinetic energy.

If any particles were left in the tube, the electrons would collide with them and be slowed down, and maximum acceleration is achieved when there is nothing for the electrons to bump into.

We need a material to produce large numbers of electrons that can then be accelerated across the glass tube; we also need a way of producing a voltage high enough to accelerate the electrons to a very high speed (i.e. to give them the large amounts of kinetic energy).

X-RAY TUBE FILAMENT

To produce the electrons a fine tungsten wire is used and twisted into a filament similar to that in a (now old-fashioned) light bulb. The tungsten is then specially treated so that passing an electric current through it to heat it will easily cause electrons to leave the surface of the metal (almost like water molecules producing steam when the water is heated). The electrons will form a sort of cloud around the filament until an additional influence is exerted (Figure 2.1).

Some of you may be thinking, 'how do the electrons do that? Aren't they supposed to push each other away? Like charges repel each other' (Chapter 1, page 7).

It's true that things are not as simple as stated earlier, additional electric supplies around the filament produce forces that keep the electrons close to the filament and in a single 'focussed', group (cloud).

Basic Guide to Dental Radiography, First Edition. Tim Reynolds.
© 2016 John Wiley & Sons, Ltd. Published 2016 by John Wiley & Sons, Ltd.

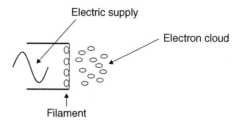

Figure 2.1 X-ray tube filament with electron cloud

From earlier statements we know that if we have a large collection of electrons, we have a large build-up of negative electric charge.

All that is needed now is for us to produce a large positive charge at the other end of the evacuated tube to attract the electrons to that end (negative charges will always want to move towards positive charges).

TRANSFORMERS

Dental intra-oral X-ray machines work at 60, 65 or 70 kV, that is, up to 70 000 V. Clearly the UK mains voltage of around 230 V must be drastically changed to reach the required level. In order to make this change, we use a transformer. A transformer (depending on how it is constructed) can be made to either increase (step up) or to decrease (step down) the voltage.

To make these transformers two wires are wound like spirals; they are called windings. The two wires form one primary winding (where the voltage comes into the system) and a secondary winding (where the voltage comes out of the system).

The arrangement shown with many windings on the primary and few on the secondary would produce a step-down transformer (the voltage exiting is smaller than that entering) (Figure 2.2).

This system with few loops on the primary and many on the secondary would give a step-up transformer (Figure 2.3).

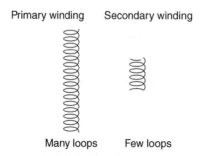

Figure 2.2 Step-down transformer windings

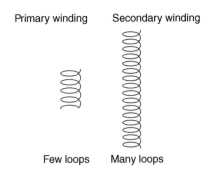

Figure 2.3 Step-up transformer windings

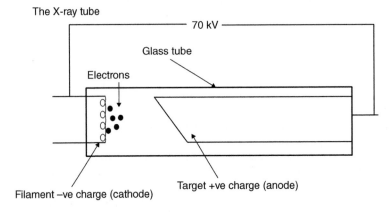

Figure 2.4 Inside the X-ray tube (tube insert)

The amount that voltage is stepped up or down is proportional to the difference between the numbers of turns of wire on each of the windings. So if there are twice as many turns on the secondary as on the primary, the voltage is doubled; for the step down half as many turns on the secondary, the voltage is halved.

The aforementioned examples give only the barest outline of how the transformer works. There are additional parts and other principles of physics, electricity and magnetism at work, but we are concerned more with the high voltage than exactly how it is produced.

The electric supply to the X-ray tube provides power to two systems at the same time (Figure 2.4):

1. It supplies low voltage to the filament at the cathode end of the tube so that it is heated to a high temperature.
2. It supplies the power to the primary winding of the large step-up transformer that is required to change the 230 V mains supply to 70 kV operating voltage.

The negatively charged filament is called the cathode and the positively charged end of the tube is the anode.

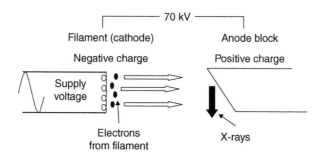

Figure 2.5 Tube current, milliamps (mA)

X-RAY TUBE ANODE

The anode (positive side) of the tube is a large copper block with a shaped end and a tungsten target set into its sloping face.

The anode is copper because during the production of X-rays, large amounts of heat are produced as a result of the process. Copper can hold large amounts of heat energy and it is a good conductor of heat.

The fact that the copper is a good conductor of heat is important because it means the heat is rapidly removed from the target area, where it is produced, to the other parts of the block, effectively making room for more heat to be put into the target area by other electrons crossing the tube.

The evacuated glass tube is not a straight tube as shown, but this model is sufficient to show the general principles of its construction and operation (Figure 2.5).

The open arrows $\Longrightarrow$ show the acceleration of the electron cloud towards the tungsten target set into the anode block. The acceleration occurs because of the 70 000 V difference between the positive and negative ends of the tube. The high voltage and the fact that the tube is a perfect vacuum (no particles for the electrons to collide with) means that the electrons reach extremely high speeds (they gain a lot of kinetic energy). These fast-moving electrons form the tube current (mA) of the X-ray machine.

The face of the anode block containing the target is shaped to ensure that the X-rays produced exit the tube roughly in the direction shown by the solid arrow ↓, it also affects the size of the X-ray focus.

VOLTAGE RECTIFICATION

We have made several references to the fact that the filament (cathode) is negative and the target (anode) is positive. The mains voltage supplying the power to our X-ray tube is however an alternating supply; this would mean that the filament and target would both be alternating between positive and negative potential. If this were allowed to occur, the electrons that we have shown flowing at high speed from the filament to the shaped target on the anode block would in fact alternate in their direction of flow.

They would sometimes flow from filament to target and sometimes from target to filament. The collision between high-speed electrons and a fine-wire filament would result in an almost immediate burnout of the filament as it could not withstand the heat generated as the electrons give up their kinetic energy.

Something has to be done to prevent connection of the filament to the positive part of the mains cycle and the anode to the negative portion. To prevent the unwanted connections, the supply to the X-ray tube is passed through a series of special gates called rectifiers. These rectifiers allow current to pass in only one direction so that by carefully rerouting the supply, we can ensure that the filament will only ever be negative and the target positive.

HALF-WAVE AND FULL-WAVE RECTIFICATION

Half-wave rectification consists of simply blocking one part of the cycle so that, for example, the positive supply is never connected to the filament (Figure 2.6).

As can be seen from this diagram, half-wave rectification completely wastes half of the electric supply. It would also mean that exposure times would have to be twice as long because you may have pushed the button during the half cycle when nothing was happening (no supply so no X-rays produced).

The waste of half the supply requires excessive exposure times (a disadvantage when it is important to eliminate patient movement). Half-wave rectification does not fit the requirements for modern X-ray equipment.

Full-wave rectification uses more rectifiers to effectively turn one part of the cycle upside down, to ensure that the filament and target are always connected to the correct electric charge, either the positive or negative side as required (Figure 2.7).

With this system both halves of the mains cycle are used so there is no wasted power and exposure times can be reduced. The one disadvantage here is that for much of the cycle, the voltage applied is much lower than the peak and would not be high enough to produce useful X-rays.

Modern X-ray equipment overcomes this problem with additional circuits that produce electric supplies that are very close or identical to the direct current that we saw delivered from a battery; these are medium- or high-frequency generators.

The graph of the supply to a modern system would look something like the one shown in Figure 2.8 with the supply showing a slight ripple around the peak value or even a direct unchanging supply such as that shown coming from a battery in Chapter 1.

Such a supply allows shorter exposure times, uses more of the available power and produces a higher number of useful X-rays.

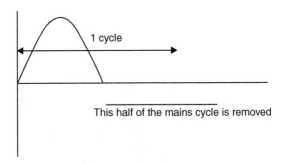

Figure 2.6 Half-wave rectified voltage waveform

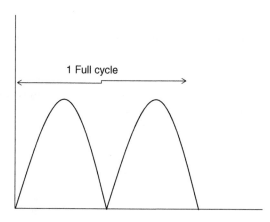

Figure 2.7 Full wave rectified voltage waveform

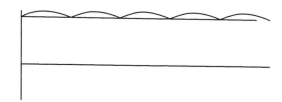

Figure 2.8 Medium- or high-frequency voltage waveform

By useful X-rays we mean those with enough energy to penetrate the tissues under investigation and produce an image on the film or digital sensor.

THE PROCESS OF X-RAY PRODUCTION

To investigate the process of X-ray production, we must go back to the infinitely small world we looked into in the first few pages of this text, the world of atomic structure deep (in atomic) terms within the target face shown in (Figure 2.9).

You will have noted that the same material (tungsten) is used for the filament and the target (X-ray producing) area of the anode.

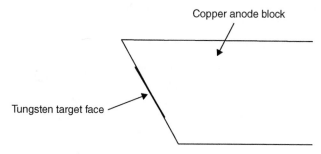

Figure 2.9 X-ray target face

The properties that make it useful for the filament are as follows: high melting point, can be drawn into a fine wire, will produce many electrons at relatively low current and does not tend to vaporise.

If the filament vaporised when heated, it would fill the tube with material and spoil the vacuum.

Similar properties make it ideal for the target. Lots of heat energy will be produced so we don't want it to reach a temperature where it will vaporise. It has high heat capacity (it can store a lot of heat with relatively low temperature rise), and it is a good conductor so much of the heat produced is taken rapidly away from the target area. These factors combine to prevent vaporisation of the target.

It also has a good conversion efficiency (produces a high number of X-rays) when absorbing kinetic energy. This good conversion efficiency is a term that is used relative to other materials. In fact only about 1–5% of the kinetic energy is converted to X-rays, and the rest is almost entirely heat; this is why heat storage and conduction are important.

Lastly tungsten can be made into a very smooth almost mirror-like surface; this helps to maximise the number of X-rays able to exit the X-ray tube.

This diagram (Figure 2.10) represents a tiny section of the sloping target face and what happens when the filament electrons make contact with it. The shapes show four atoms in the tungsten, the solid inner circle being the nucleus with a large number of protons; there will be 74 in each nucleus because the atomic number of tungsten is 74. This means there will be a significant positive charge in each nucleus.

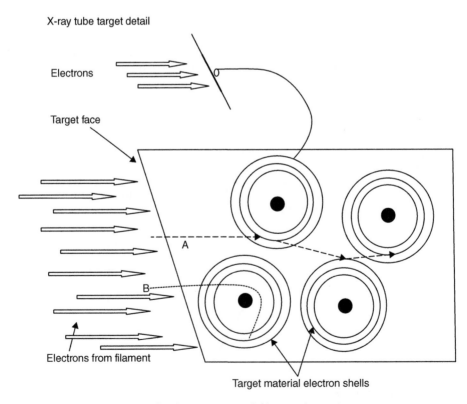

Figure 2.10 Tungsten target detail (interactions with filament electrons)

The three larger circles surrounding the nucleus represent the K, L and M electron shells; there will of course be many more shells than this as 74 electrons could not fit into just three. (We will call these target electrons.) The four atoms shown are deep (in atomic terms) within the target.

The filament electrons shown approaching the sloping face of the target material will interact with the particles in the target; the nature of that interaction will determine how many X-rays, if any, will be produced, the level of energy they will possess and the amount of heat that is produced.

It is not possible nor necessary to show all potential interactions between the electrons accelerated across the tube and the target material; we simply need to show two of the major possibilities.

The dashed line, _ _ _ _ _ _, labelled A shows the path of a filament electron that will interact with an outer shell 'target electron'; the interaction causes the filament electron to give up some of its energy and to continue through the material with a slightly changed direction. The electron that has crossed the X-ray tube and entered the target may go through a large number of such interactions before giving up all of the kinetic energy it gained from the 70 kV applied to the tube.

During these interactions the target electrons may be temporarily raised to another electron shell level (this is excitation), or they may be removed from the atom altogether (ionisation).

This type of interaction will produce large amounts of heat but very few, 'if any', useful X-rays.

The dotted line, ▪▪▪▪▪▪▪▪▪▪▪▪▪▪▪▪, labelled B shows the path of a filament electron that enters the target and passes close to a nucleus. The large positive charge of the nucleus exerts a strong force of attraction on the electron and its path changes dramatically. This large change in direction results in the electron giving up much of its kinetic energy, and causes a large change in its velocity (speed) it is slowed down considerably.

This second type of interaction is much more likely to produce X-rays. The energy of the X-rays could be anything from the maximum 70 kV down to single figures; this will depend on the deflection (change in direction) of the electron. As the angle of deflection increases, the energy released also increases. If a 70 kV 'filament electron' was completely brought to rest in a single interaction, it could produce X-rays with energy of 70 kV.

Although we have shown the filament electron marked B producing X-rays at the first target atom that it approaches this may not be the case. Filament electrons may go through several minor interactions in the target before eventually undergoing a major interaction and producing X-ray photons. The amount of energy available for conversion to X-rays is lower because some has been given up in the earlier interactions.

The X-rays produced in this way are called bremsstrahlung radiation (literally braking radiation) because they are produced by the slowing down of the accelerated filament electron.

Not all of those electrons passing close to the nucleus will produce X-rays.

- NB: Remember that the electrons are not converted to X-rays. It is the kinetic energy (energy of movement) they possess as a result of their acceleration that is converted. The electrons are still part of the circuit and may go around again and produce more X-rays.
- This is rather like the water in a fountain. The pump pushes it high into the air where it has potential energy. It falls gaining kinetic energy that is changed to sound and a little heat as it hits the main body of water. Sound and heat have been produced from the kinetic energy but the water still exists to be circulated again.

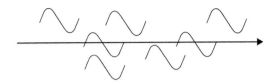

Figure 2.11 Individual X-ray quanta forming a beam

The X-rays emitted from the target do not form a constant stream like water coming from a tap; they are more like tennis balls being fired from a machine used for training.

The reason for this is partly that all of the electrons do not produce X-rays so there will be gaps (not exactly how it occurs but a good way to think of it).

Although oversimplified this idea of X-ray production allows us to introduce an important point about X-rays. As already stated the X-rays do not form a constant stream but are individual tiny 'packets' of energy called quanta or photons. From this point quantum will refer to a single 'packet' of X-ray energy, and quanta will refer to a beam containing a number of them. When talking about imaging we will refer simply to the X-ray beam, it will contain billions of quanta (Figure 2.11).

The bremsstrahlung radiation is also called continuous spectra. The individual quanta will have a level of energy equal (or similar) to the kinetic energy lost by the electron when the quantum was produced. A beam of continuous spectra will have quanta with a large range of energy levels because some 'filament electrons' will give up all of their energy in a single interaction where others may give it up gradually through several.

Remember that the closer a 'filament electron' passes to the large positive charge of the nucleus, the greater the proportion of its kinetic energy it gives up.

BREMSSTRAHLUNG (CONTINUOUS) SPECTRA

A graph showing the range of energy and number of quanta emerging from the X-ray tube is shown in Figure 2.12. The curved line represents the continuous spectrum.

The point marked X is the maximum energy of any quantum; it will be equal to the kV selected on the X-ray machine. These quanta would be produced if there was massive slowing of the electron hitting the target so that it gave up all of its energy in one go and that energy produced an X-ray quantum.

There are a number of factors that could change the exact shape of this graph, but for this basic understanding we do not need to investigate these factors.

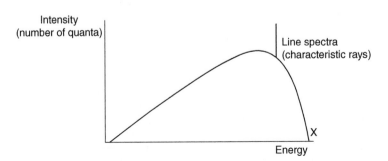

Figure 2.12 Distribution of continuous and line spectra

X-RAY PRODUCTION

We do however need to talk about the additional line of the graph labelled line spectra or characteristic rays.

The two names are in fact purely descriptive terms.

Line spectra should be fairly obvious from looking at the graph, the quanta all have exactly the same energy and the intensity is shown as a single straight vertical line.

The term characteristic rays is not obvious at all; it comes from the fact that the energy of these quanta is specific to the target material and a specific electron shell within the atoms of the target material. (That is to say, it is *characteristic* of those two factors.) Changing the target material or the electron shell in the target material that the filament electron interacts with will change the energy of the emitted quantum.

PRODUCTION OF LINE SPECTRA

The diagram (Figure 2.13) shows an electron crossing the X-ray tube and interacting with a K shell electron in the target material. The K shell electron is removed from its shell and moves off through the target; the filament electron also continues through the target in a new direction.

On page 3 of Chapter 1, we discussed the fact that electrons could not be placed in an outer shell until inner shells were filled and that if an outer shell electron moves down to fill an inner shell gap; it has to give up some of its energy.

This is exactly what happens in the X-ray tube target when characteristic rays are produced. We have shown a K shell electron being ejected and the gap being filled by an L shell electron. The L shell electron has to give up energy in doing this and this energy could be given up as a **characteristic ray**.

Its energy is 'characteristic' of the L to K shell energy difference in tungsten. We said previously that the electron shells in a solid are in fact bands due to the influence of other atoms. This means that not all K shell or L shell electrons have exactly the same energy. Characteristic emissions reflect this in that there will not be a single K 'characteristic' line as shown in the diagram. In tungsten the K lines will be in a range just below to just above 60 kV M to L and N to M and other characteristic rays may be produced.

Any beam of X-ray quanta will consist of continuous spectra with a wide energy range and line spectra with a single specific energy level.

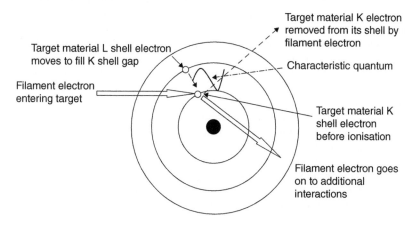

Figure 2.13 Production of characteristic (line) spectra

FACTORS AFFECTING THE NUMBER OF X-RAY QUANTA PRODUCED

The number of X-ray quanta produced will depend on a number of factors; these factors are what we commonly refer to as exposure.

Exposure is made up of three parts, two of which we have already discussed but not in terms of exposure factors.

The potential of 70 000 V set between the cathode (filament) and the anode (target) is called the kVp (kilovolts peak). The lower case p represents peak, because we always refer to the maximum (peak) value of the potential applied across an X-ray tube.

If the kV is raised, the filament electrons (as we have so far called them) will be attracted towards the target by a greater force, and they will be given more kinetic energy (will travel faster). If the filament electrons have greater kinetic energy, the probability that their interactions with target material will produce X-rays is increased.

Increasing kVp will give us X-ray quanta with a maximum energy equal to the new kVp; it will also produce more X-ray quanta at each of the energy levels found within the bremsstrahlung spectrum.

Overall the number of X-ray quanta is proportional to kVp^2.

The electrons accelerated across the X-ray tube that we have been calling filament electrons do in fact produce an electric current (charge moving between two points in a circuit is current). The two points we are moving charge between are the filament and the target (cathode and anode).

This is called the 'tube current' and like all currents it is measured in amps. The amp is a relatively large current and X-ray tube currents are small, measured in thousandths of an amp. Dental X-ray machines usually work on 8–10 mA (8–10 thousandths of an amp).

If you double the number of electrons crossing the X-ray tube, you double the number of interactions with target atoms and double the number of X-ray quanta produced. The intensity (number of quanta) is therefore directly proportional to the mA. Triple the mA gives approximately three times as many X-ray quanta.

The third factor that makes up our expression of exposure is time. If the exposure time is doubled, the tube current will be flowing for twice as long and double the number of electrons will have crossed the X-ray tube. Just as doubling the tube current gives twice as many interactions and twice as many X-ray quanta; the same will happen when we double the exposure time.

So doubling the exposure time will produce twice as many X-ray quanta. We call the product of mA and exposure time milliamp seconds (mA s).

10 mA × 1 s would be 10 mA s, and 10 mA for 2 s would be 20 mA s; of course exposure time in dental intra-oral examinations is measured in only fractions of a second, typically 0.12 s.

In summary changing any of the exposure factors, kVp, mA or exposure time will have an effect on the number of X-ray quanta produced. The greatest effect will be produced by kVp because intensity is proportional to kVp^2.

The kVp will also affect the, maximum and average energies of the beam. The increase in the average energy of the beam makes it more able to penetrate matter; the beam is said to be harder. This increase in beam hardness has implications for the type of image that will be produced and for the radiation protection of the patient.

THE PROPERTIES OF X-RAYS

X-rays are part of the electromagnetic spectrum; this range of radiations includes radio waves, microwaves, visible light, X-rays, gamma rays and cosmic rays. Radio waves are low-energy radiation, light somewhere in the middle and X-rays towards the top of the total range of energies.

They all share the same general physical properties: they are electromagnetic radiations, and they all therefore have both an electric element and a magnetic element. The two elements (electric and magnetic) have a wave nature similar to the one we used to show alternating voltage and current, that is, a sinusoidal waveform. The electric and magnetic waves lie and move at right angles to each other (Figure 2.14).

A feature of electricity that we did not discuss previously is that if you have an electric current flowing in a conductor, there will also be a magnetic field. Similarly if you move a magnet close to or within an electrical conductor, you will get an induced voltage, and if there is a complete circuit, a current will flow.

This is called electromagnetic induction.

If you studied combined sciences or physics at some point in the past, you may have conducted a simple experiment to show this phenomenon (Figure 2.15).

Pushing the magnet into the coil of wire will cause the meter needle to flick in one direction; pulling the magnet out will cause the meter needle to flick in the other direction. By constantly pushing it in and out, you could set up your own alternating voltage and current.

If you put the magnet into the coil and leave it there, nothing happens as it is the movement that produces the voltage. If you place a piece of steel into the coil and pass a current through the coil, the steel will become magnetic. In fact even without the steel in place, there would be a magnetic force; the steel just intensifies it.

X-RAY PRODUCTION

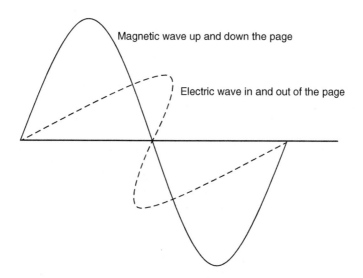

Figure 2.14 Electromagnetic radiations (configuration of electric and magnetic waves)

X-RAY PRODUCTION

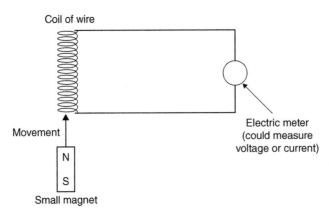

Coil of wire

Movement

N

S

Small magnet

Electric meter
(could measure
voltage or current)

Figure 2.15 Electromagnetic induction

So moving magnets will induce voltage and current and moving current will induce magnetism. This is exactly the situation we have in a quantum of X-radiation. There is a moving electric and moving magnetic element making up the whole thing. These two elements are able (effectively) to create each other and they are therefore mutually supportive (each one props up the other). This means that unlike most waves they do not simply die out; they will go on forever unless they are acted on by another force that uses up their energy.

X-ray quanta hitting electrons or interacting with the nucleus in any material will cause the quanta to lose energy, and if there are enough such interactions, they will be totally absorbed and will cease to exist.

This could of course take some considerable time, and they are able to travel large distances even in solid materials (remember that all atoms are mostly free space; there are few solid particles).

This becomes very important when we come to considering what would be considered to be a safe area to stand in if the only material in the path of the beam is air.

In a vacuum the X-ray quanta will go on forever because the electric and magnetic elements support each other and there are no solid particles to cause the collisions that would absorb their energy.

The list of properties of X-rays has not really changed since Wilhelm Conrad Roentgen first completed his experiments. Some of these features will not match perfectly with modern concepts in physics, but they are sufficient for our purposes:

Travel in straight lines. This is a big reason for us being able to produce reasonably accurate images with them. They travel from our X-ray tube past the edge of an object and on to our image recorder giving us a number of image points that are in the same place relative to each other as they are in the original object. If the X-ray quanta followed curved pathways, no accurate image could ever be produced (Figure 2.16).

- When the X-ray photons travel in straight lines, the position that they will strike the film can be predicted and an image is formed. If the photons followed a random curved path, features of the object could be placed anywhere randomly on the film (dashed line) Figure 2.16.

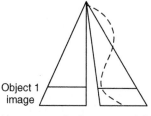

Here we see the image we might
expect with X-rays travelling in
straight lines

Figure 2.16 X-rays travelling in straight lines

Obey the inverse square law. This means that the intensity of an X-ray beam varies inversely with the square of the distance from the source. That sounds a bit complicated so let us break it down.

X-ray beam intensity (number of quanta in a particular area) varies inversely (gets smaller) with the square of the distance from the source (multiply the distance 'double, triple, etc.' by itself to get the exact relationship between the two intensities).

This gives us

$$I \propto \frac{1}{d^2} \quad \text{or} \quad I \propto \frac{1}{4} \quad \text{if distance is doubled } d^2 \text{ is } 2 \times 2 \quad I = \text{intensity of the beam}$$

or

$$I \propto \frac{1}{9} \quad \text{if distance is trebled.}$$

Simply put, if you move twice the distance from the source, you get a quarter of the dose, and if you move three times the distance, you get a ninth of the dose per square centimetre. This is because the beam spreads out as it gets further from its origin and less of it hits whatever has been put into its path (including people). This inverse square law is an important concept for the protection of staff and other people not actually having an X-ray examination.

As with all things in science, it's not quite as easy as that because the law is only true if the X-ray origin is an infinitely small point source and that the beam is travelling in a vacuum. Having said that it remains true that when considering safety, distance is important; there is potential for very big dose reductions for staff by making sure you are at the maximum distance you can be from a source of radiation.

Penetrate matter. X-ray quanta are effectively tiny packets of energy. When we say tiny in this instance, we mean even in relation to the very small particles, like electrons, that we have discussed previously. This means in simple terms they are able to slip through the spaces between the solid particles that make up the atoms and molecules that are the building blocks of our world.

Many people make the mistake that any old piece of lead will absorb any X-rays that come into contact with it. This is not so; the amount of absorption depends on both the beam energy and the thickness of lead in its path. If lead protection is too thin, many X-ray quanta will be able to pass through it.

Cause excitation. We have mentioned excitation briefly when talking about electrons crossing the X-ray tube and interacting with target material electrons. Although the excitation process is similar, we must not mix up the two interactions. In this case we are talking about X-ray quanta interacting with electrons in any material.

The electron that is hit by or simply has a quantum pass close by will be given energy by the quantum. This energy causes the electron to be raised to a higher energy level, because with the additional energy it can no longer remain in its original shell. Soon after the quantum has passed by, the elevated (excited) electron will give up the additional energy it was given and will return to its original orbit, or it may settle in a higher orbit if its original place has been taken by an electron from further out.

Excitation causes only a temporary small rise in temperature; there is no permanent change to the contents or the structure of the atom.

Cause ionisation. Again we briefly mentioned ionisation in target material interactions with filament electrons, and the process of ionisation is similar in that case and with X-ray interactions with matter. Ionisation completely removes an electron from its shell and from the atom. The shell will be filled by an electron from a shell further out; eventually there will be no more shells to donate an electron, and a space will exist on the outer shell. Remember that these outer shell electrons give the atom its chemical properties (they give it the ability to make bonds with other atoms). Ionisation therefore changes the chemical structure and reactivity of the atom. Also, as each electron changes from an outer to an inner shell, it will have to give up some of its energy.

There are a number of important properties of X-ray that arise from their ability to ionise or excite atoms:

Biological effect. X-ray quanta will cause permanent changes to biological tissues; these changes can be fatal.

Chemical effect. They will cause changes to chemical substances and may actually change it from one form to another; this fact can be used to measure radiation doses.

Photographic effect. They will cause a reaction in a photographic emulsion, so that when processed we can see increased density (the plate turns black). This was one of the observations that led Roentgen to develop the theories of their diagnostic use. It is still the method of recording for many radiographic images.

Fluoroscopic effect. The quanta will make some crystals glow; this is due to the absorption of X-ray photons. This effect is used in the intensifying screens in OPG cassettes as a way of reducing the dose delivered to the patient. High-energy X-ray photons are absorbed and produce a much larger number of low-energy light photons.

They travel at the speed of light. This is 3×10^8 m/s (i.e. 300 million metres).

They are unaffected by electric or magnetic fields. This does not seem possible as X-ray quanta themselves have both an electric and magnetic force. Any electric or magnetic field will interact with any other electric or magnetic field it comes into close contact with. However within the general field of use, the X-rays that we employ do not come into contact with fields with enough strength to alter their behaviour.

They cannot be detected by any of the human senses. You can't see, feel, taste or smell X-ray quanta.

Chapter 3

X-ray interaction with matter

Whenever X-rays pass through any material, there are three possible outcomes:

1. They may pass through, completely unchanged.
2. They may pass through in altered form (new direction and lower energy).
3. They may be completely absorbed by the material and not emerge at all.

All of these outcomes are possible in any material other than a vacuum. In a vacuum only the first option (pass through unchanged) will occur. This is because the second and third – pass through with lower energy and in a new direction or not pass through at all – occur because the X-ray quanta interact with the solid particles (nucleus or orbiting electrons) within the material. A vacuum of course has none of these particles, so the X-ray quanta pass through completely unhindered and unchanged.

In all other materials (media), there will be particles for the quanta to interact with, and the number of such interactions will depend on specific factors, most of which will alter the number of solid particles in the path of the X-ray beam and another factor that changes the way in which the beam interacts when it does come into contact with those particles.

How is it possible for X-ray quanta to pass through materials other than a vacuum completely unchanged? Surely in any reasonably solid object the quanta are bound to come into contact with solid particles.

To understand why the previous statement is not correct, we need to look back into our atom and investigate its structure further.

It is not possible to represent in a diagram the true scale of atomic radius (the distance between the outer edges of the outer electron shells) compared with the volume of solid particles present in the atom. If we look back to pages 3 and 4, we talked about the amount of free space (gaps between solid particles) in atoms. It is suggested, to illustrate this that the solid particles contained within the average person would fit on the head of a pin. This fact alone indicates that there must be some pretty wide open gaps.

Add to this the fact that the X-ray quanta are tiny even compared with a single electron, and there is a lot of room for these tiny quanta to pass through the gaps in even materials that we consider to be very solid (such as lead).

As a demonstration, imagine that you put a hula hoop on the floor to represent the K shell of a material and put two grape pips somewhere on the hoop to be the two K shell

Basic Guide to Dental Radiography, First Edition. Tim Reynolds.
© 2016 John Wiley & Sons, Ltd. Published 2016 by John Wiley & Sons, Ltd.

electrons. Place an orange in the middle to be the nucleus, and then throw a single strawberry seed at the whole construction.

What do you think the chances of the strawberry seed hitting the orange or grape pips are?

The actual atomic sizes are even more immense than this example, but it gives you some idea of the chances of collisions occurring.

The number of quanta passing through a material with little or no change is one of the facts that we will be considering when talking about where it is safe to stand during an X-ray examination.

When looking at the journey of a single quantum passing through a material, the chances of it interacting with any particle are very small.

One reason for this is the amount of empty space in the atom, and the other is that everything is moving. This means a quantum, even if it is on a similar path to a circulating electron, has to arrive at exactly the same time and place as the electron to interact with it.

Despite this low probability many quanta do hit something, simply because of the total number of quanta contained in any beam. Even in the lowest intra-oral dose you can give, there will be billions of quanta.

Interactions between the quanta and particles in the material ensure that less X-ray quanta will come out of the material than entered it. This process is called **attenuation** and it is defined in the following way.

> • Attenuation of a beam of radiation is the fractional reduction in beam intensity as it passes through any material other than a vacuum.

The beam entering a material is called the incident beam and that exiting the material is called the transmitted beam.

Intensity is the number of quanta found in (or crossing through) a particular area, so if we draw two squares of the same size and place 10 quanta in one and 5 in the other, the intensity in the second box will be half of that in the first. If we call the boxes 1 unit of area, then the intensity of the first is 10 to 1 and in the second 5 to 1 (Figure 3.1).

If you pass more X-ray quanta through any area, there will be more chance of those quanta interacting with particles in the material that they pass through. This is important when considering X-rays passing through human tissue and the effect they may have as they do so.

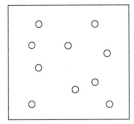

Box of 1 unit area
Intensity 10 to 1

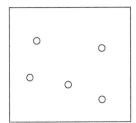

Box of 1 unit area
Intensity 5 to 1

Figure 3.1 Intensity of a beam of X-rays

FACTORS AFFECTING ATTENUATION

In this example there are eight quanta in the incident beam and two in the transmitted, so three quarters of them do not come through the material; this means there is 75% attenuation (Figure 3.2).

The second example shows an attenuation factor of only 50%, considerably less than the first (Figure 3.3).

When considering what could account for this difference, we have to look for factors that could put more solid particles into the path of the quanta in the first situation.

When talking about atomic structures, we found that different materials have a different, specific number of protons in the nucleus; this is defined by the atomic number. The atomic number also gives some idea of the number of electrons in orbits around the nucleus. It is also an indicator of the total number of particles in an atom because the greater the number of protons, the greater the number of neutrons.

If we see two pieces of material that look the same and are exactly the same size but the attenuation is different, we could make the assumption that the material with the higher attenuation value has a higher atomic number.

This high atomic number would place more particles per atom in the path of the beam of X-rays. So we conclude that the material producing 75% (Figure 3.2)

X-RAY INTERACTION WITH MATTER

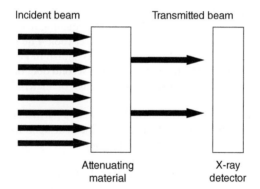

Figure 3.2 Attenuation of an X-ray beam (75% attenuation)

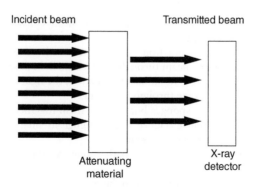

Figure 3.3 Attenuation of an X-ray beam (50% attenuation)

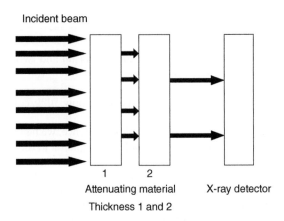

Incident beam

1   2
Attenuating material   X-ray detector
Thickness 1 and 2

Figure 3.4 Attenuation of an X-ray beam (thickness of the attenuator)

attenuation has a higher atomic number than the one producing 50% (Figure 3.3) attenuation. We are mainly considering the number of electrons as each atom has only one nucleus.

What happens if we add more of the same attenuation material?

When looking at the addition of new layers of attenuating material, it would be easy to make the mistaken assumption that if the first layer took 4 quanta out of 8, then the second layer would take the other 4 leaving none. As shown in Figure 3.4, this does not happen; the first layer gave 50% attenuation and the second does the same so two quanta eventually hit the detector. If we added another later of material, then one quantum would hit the detector.

The general rule then says that each new thickness of a particular attenuating material would remove the same percentage of the quanta incident upon its surface. This rule is only true if the general nature of the beam of radiation (range of energies of individual quanta) remains constant.

What actually happens is that in the first layer the lower energy quanta are absorbed more easily and the higher energy ones that are left are more penetrating, so the attenuation will be slightly lower in the second layer. This is because the average energy of the quanta in the beam is higher after it has passed through the first layer of attenuating material.

We often find a mismatch between the purely scientific consideration of a situation and what is actually found in practice.

A third factor affecting attenuation can be examined using a simple household object – imagine passing X-ray beam through a 2 inch thick bath sponge (Figure 3.5a).

No surprise to see that there is not much attenuation; the figures show only 25%, and three quarters of the quanta come through the sponge.

What if we add three more sponges but squeeze them together so that the beam still passes through 2 inches of sponge (Figure 3.5b) a higher attenuation is seen.

What has caused the difference in attenuation?

We are still passing the beam through bath sponge so the atomic number has not changed.

We have squeezed the sponges together, so there is still 2 inches of sponge, so thickness has not changed.

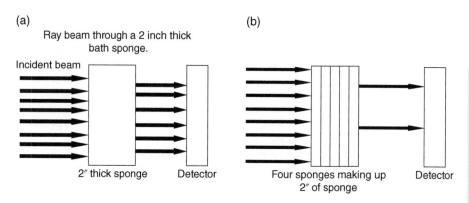

Figure 3.5 Attenuation of an X-ray beam (density of the attenuator): (a) 2 inch thick sponge and (b) four sponges making up 2 inches of sponge

We have however changed the density; the solid particles in the sponge are pushed closer together, so there is less space for the quanta to pass through unhindered.

Three features of the attenuating material then can affect the level of attenuation seen:

1. Atomic number
2. Thickness
3. Density

The factors affecting attenuation are also the factors that will create our radiographic image. This is because, as the beam passes through areas where atomic number, thickness or density is different, the number of X-rays passing through to the film or sensor will be changed.

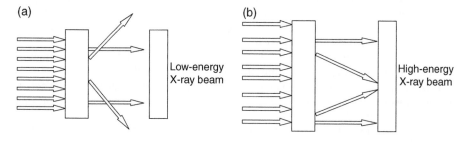

Figure 3.6 Attenuation of an X-ray beam: (a) low beam energy and (b) high beam energy

If we pass a beam of X-rays through two identical attenuators, atomic number, thickness and density being the same, there may still be a difference in attenuation.

In this case it is the nature of the beam that is different; the attenuation will be changed by an increase or decrease in the average energy of the individual quanta in the beam.

Figure 3.6a and b, each show eight quanta hitting the attenuator with four coming through to the other side. Of the four shown coming through, two pass straight through and two come through at a different angle of travel to the path they entered on.

In Figure 3.6a, the two quanta that come through with a new direction of travel are missing the detector. This would mean that although they have passed through the attenuator, we don't know that they have done so, and as a result they are included in the total attenuation (they are missing from the intensity at the detector).

In Figure 3.6b the two quanta on a new path still hit the detector and will not be included in the attenuation figure.

The quanta we are considering are scattered by their interaction with the particles in the material. The difference in the attenuation is not about how much scatter is produced but about the direction that the scatter takes.

Higher-energy beams produce narrow-angle scatter (its path is close to that of the incident quantum). Low-energy beams produce wide-angle scatter (where the new path is far from that of the incident quantum).

The effect of the beam energy on the angle of scatter not only affects the attenuation but has important implications for radiation protection.

The previous two examples have attenuation figures of 75% Figure 3.6a and 50% (Figure 3.6b); in each case there are quanta that we have not taken into account. We have shown two quanta coming straight through and two being scattered, in each case leaving four to be explained. The four we have not explained are part of the total attenuation because they have not come through the material, but what has happened to them?

The scattered quanta have collided with something that provides enough of a barrier to remove some but not all of their energy, and to knock them off their original path, they still exist but have a new direction of travel and reduced energy.

The other quanta that are part of the attenuation have much more serious collisions with particles in the attenuating material and give up all of their energy in the interaction, the quanta ceasing to exist (they have been absorbed).

Total attenuation consists therefore of two parts, **absorption** and **scatter**, but what determines which process the quanta go through?

Once again we have to think about the structure of the atom to explain why each of these interactions may occur.

When talking about electron orbits, we said that electrons in outer shells have higher energy than those that occupy inner shells, and if electrons move from an outer shell to an inner shell, they have to give up some of their energy because they must have the right amount of energy to exist in any particular shell.

We don't need to know the exact nature of this electron energy, but it is important to remember that it gets higher as we move to shells further from the nucleus.

It will help you to remember if you think of this energy in the same way as the potential energy gained by an object as you lift it from the floor to a low shelf and then moving it to a higher shelf.

If we imagine that all electrons start at the nucleus and have to be moved out to their shells, it helps to remind us that the outer shell will have greater energy.

The nucleus has a large concentration of positive charge; if you move an electron from beside the nucleus to the K shell, you have to do work to pull it against the attraction of that positive charge. The positive charge of the protons in the nucleus attracts the electrons because the electrons have a negative charge. This is like lifting an item from the floor to a low shelf: you are doing work against the force of gravity and the potential energy of the body is equal to the work done in lifting the item to that shelf.

Electrons in the K shell then can be thought of as having energy equal to the work done in moving electrons from the nucleus to the K shell.

If we then move an electron to the L shell, we have to do work to get it as far as the K shell and then more work to move it on to the L shell Figure 3.7. Overall we will have

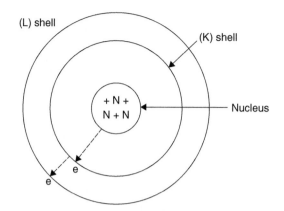

Figure 3.7 Electron energy in successive electron shells

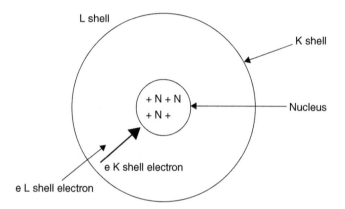

Figure 3.8 Binding energy in successive electron shells

done more work getting an electron to the L shell than the K shell. This is like lifting an item to a low shelf from the floor then onto a higher shelf. The item will have more potential on the higher shelf, and the electron in the L shell will have higher electron energy than one in the K shell.

There is however another type of energy we need to think of; it is called binding energy (Figure 3.8).

The arrows indicate the force of attraction exerted by the nucleus on the orbiting electrons.

The binding energy tells us how much energy we would need to remove an electron from its shell and from the atom (how much work would we need to do). The concentration of positive charge in the nucleus exerts force of attraction on the electrons. If an electron lies in the K shell, this force is very strong because the electron is close to the positive charge.

When we move the electron to the L shell, it is much further from the positive charge of the protons, and the force of attraction between them is much lower. It would therefore take a much lower input of energy to remove an L shell electron from the atom than it would a K shell electron.

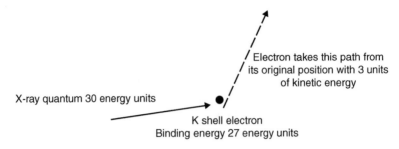

Electron takes this path from
its original position with 3 units
of kinetic energy

X-ray quantum 30 energy units

K shell electron
Binding energy 27 energy units

Figure 3.9 Photoelectric absorption

Two types of energy then are connected to electrons: binding energy that is high in inner shell and low in outer ones and electron energy that is low in inner shells and high in outer shells.

The difference in binding energy between inner and outer shells explains why some of the quanta that interact with a material are scattered and others are absorbed.

In order to explain exactly what happens, I am going to use some simple numbers that will be easy to follow but bear absolutely no relationship to the actual numbers in practice

Photoelectric absorption of quanta occurs when the quantum entering the material has an energy level that is equal to or only slightly higher than the binding energy of the electron that it interacts with.

When this type of interaction occurs, the quantum hits an inner shell electron and expels it from the atom (ionisation). Because the quantum has a level of energy that is only just enough to overcome the binding energy of the electron, it gives all of it up in removing the electron from the shell and pushing it out of the limits of the atom. In order to expel the electron from the atom, the quantum must give the electron a certain amount of kinetic energy (energy of movement) in order for it to travel to the border of the atom and beyond.

Now for the imaginary numbers. Let us give the X-ray quantum 30 units of energy and cause it to collide with a K shell electron that has a binding energy of 27 units of energy. Clearly here the quantum does have more energy than the electron has binding energy but not much (Figure 3.9).

In this example the quantum gives up 27 of its 30 energy units to simply remove the electron from its shell; it gives up the remaining 3 in giving the electron enough energy to exit the atom. This means that removing the electron first from its shell and then from the atom, the quantum has given up all of its 30 units of energy and it therefore no longer exists (it has been completely absorbed).

This type of interaction is photoelectric absorption. It is the most significant attenuation process for X-ray beams up to an energy level of 70 kV. It is therefore the primary attenuation process for many intra-oral dental X-ray machines.

Scattering could be one of two types.

Classical scatter occurs when the incoming quantum interacts in a minor way with an outer shell electron (effectively, just brushes it). In this type of interaction, there is little change to the quantum; it has given up only a small part of its energy, and it continues on almost the same path as it arrived on. We are not much concerned with this type of scatter.

Compton scatter occurs when the incoming quantum interacts in a major way (large collision) with an electron in the material. Compton scatter will take place if this incoming

X-RAY INTERACTION WITH MATTER

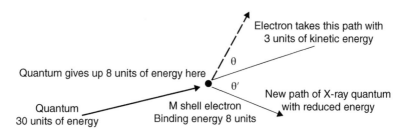

Figure 3.10 Compton scattering

quantum has a level of energy much greater than the binding energy of the electron that it hits. The electron will be expelled from the atom (ionisation), but instead of being absorbed completely, the quantum continues with a reduced level of energy and in a new direction.

Remember these figures are for illustration only and the levels of energy indicated are entirely fictitious.

Assume the quantum has a level of energy equal to 30 units and it interacts with an electron with a binding energy of 8 units (outer shell electron). Clearly the quantum has much more energy than that required to remove the electron from its orbit and to expel it from the atom (Figure 3.10).

The quantum after the collision will have energy equal to the original quantum (30) minus the binding energy of the electron (8) and the kinetic energy it was given (3), so the quantum continues with an energy level of 19 units. The electron (Compton recoil electron) path and the new quantum path at are exactly the same angle in relation to the original quantum path ($\theta = \theta'$).

The amount of kinetic energy gained by the recoil electron and lost by the quantum is proportional to the angle of scatter of the electron and the quantum.

Compton scattering becomes the predominant scattering process once beam energy exceeds 70 kV; this would seem quite logical as the higher the beam energy, the more likely it is that quantum energy will be much greater than the binding energy of any electron that it comes into contact with.

Compton is much more likely when the interaction takes place between an incoming quantum and an electron in one of the shells further from the nucleus (binding energy will be low).

Don't think that below 70 kV you will have photoelectric absorption and above you will have Compton. They overlap; it's just that each is predominant at different energy levels.

Chapter 4

Principles of image formation

What we are trying to achieve with our radiograph is an image that looks as close as possible to a perfect copy of the object we are targeting for the examination. A radiograph is the correct name for the image; many people call them X-rays, but X-rays are the packets of energy that come from the X-ray tube (you can't see them).

In trying to achieve our aim we have to remember that what we are producing is a simple shadow image; try shining a torch at any complex object and see how good the resulting image is when compared with the original object.

Because of the difficulties of the image being this simple shadow picture, we have to do all that we can to make it as good an image as we possibly can.

To start thinking about this we need to consider something called imaging geometry. I know people didn't enjoy geometry at school, but all we are talking about here is the equivalent of shining that torch at an object.

IMAGING GEOMETRY

To produce an absolutely perfect image, all of the following must be in place:

The X-ray quanta must originate from an infinitely small point source.
The distance from the X-ray source to the object under examination must be relatively long.
The distance from the source to the film/sensor plate must be relatively long.
The distance from the object to the film/sensor must be relatively short.
The central part of the X-ray beam must be perpendicular to the object and film/sensor.
The central part of the beam must be directed at the centre of the object and centre of the film/sensor.
The film/sensor must be parallel to the object under examination.

    The X-ray source is generally referred to as the focus.
    Distance from focus to object is focus-to-object distance (FOD).
    Distance from focus to film/sensor is focus-to-film distance (FFD).
    Distance from object to film/sensor is object-to-film distance (OFD).

Basic Guide to Dental Radiography, First Edition. Tim Reynolds.
© 2016 John Wiley & Sons, Ltd. Published 2016 by John Wiley & Sons, Ltd.

If all of the above factors are in place, the image will be perfect. It will not surprise you to learn that it is a virtually impossible task.

The requirement in fact falls apart at the first statement – the X-rays cannot originate from an infinitely small point source; if they did it would mean focussing the fast-moving filament electrons onto a tiny spec of the target area.

If this was the case, we would destroy the target each time we used it. This is because of the massive amount of heat generated by the majority of interactions between the filament electrons and target material.

If all of that heat was focussed onto one small area, the temperature rise would be such that the target material would start to vaporise, destroying the vacuum that we need in the tube and eventually totally destroying the target.

To reduce this temperature rise, we have to spread the heat loading over a greater area of the target. Electrons crossing the tube must be focussed onto a relatively large area so no one part is subject to too much heat input.

We said previously that the shape of the target face helps to ensure that the X-rays are emitted in the correct direction; another reason for the shape is the need to reduce the temperature rise during the exposure.

We need the focus to be as small as possible because a smaller focus gives an image with better resolution (more fine detail can be seen).

The diagram on the left of Figure 4.1 shows the target area (focus) that we need for the image to show us the right level of fine detail. If we accelerated all of filament electrons (mA) towards this small area (apparent target area), the temperature rise would be greater than the target material could withstand.

Instead of doing this we accelerate the electrons towards a target area that is the size of that shown in the diagram on the right of figure 4.1. Increasing the area means that the total heat input to the target is spread over a wider area (actual target area) and this reduces the temperature rise in each small area during the exposure to a more manageable level. We still need the X-rays to come from an area (focus) of similar size to that shown on the left.

The two requirements seem to be impossible to achieve.

Spreading the heat over a large area without increasing the size of the focus is achieved by the slope of the target face (Figure 4.2).

The large rectangular area that the filament electrons hit and where the X-rays originate is called the actual focus. The smaller area that it appears the X-rays originate from (when viewed along the line of the emerging beam) is called the apparent focus.

The importance of the apparent focus is that a radiographic image cannot demonstrate clearly any structure that is smaller than the apparent focus; this is a fact of simple geometry (Figure 4.3).

PRINCIPLES OF IMAGE FORMATION

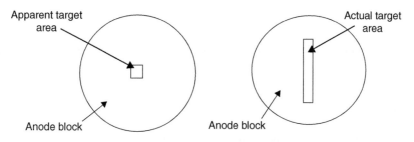

Figure 4.1 Apparent and actual (line) focus

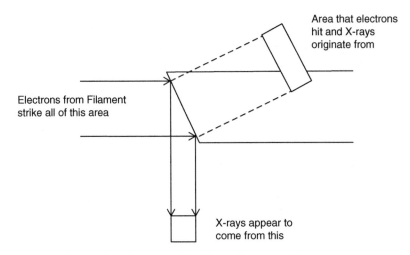

Figure 4.2 Production of small apparent focus from a large actual focus

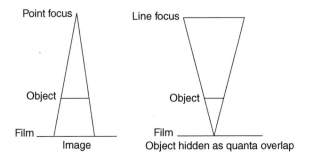

Figure 4.3 Effect of focus size on fine detail

As can be seen when the X-rays come from a point source, they pass the edges of the object and produce a good sharp image on the film. When the X-rays come from a line focus larger than the object, the X-ray quanta from the edges of the focus pass the edges of the object and meet at the same point on the film. The object in the second case will have disappeared from the image.

THE IDEAL IMAGING SYSTEM

Everything required for a perfectly accurate image (Figure 4.4) is included in this example:

Relatively long FFD and FOD.
Relatively short OFD.
Film and object parallel to each other.
Central X-rays are perpendicular to the film and object.
Central X-rays directed to the middle of the film and object.
X-rays originate from a point source.

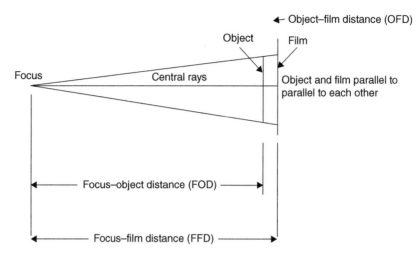

Figure 4.4 Ideal imaging geometry

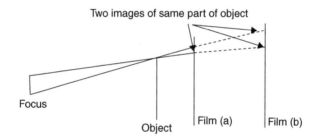

Figure 4.5 Effect of focus on blurring of the image

We have already described why the X-rays cannot come from a point source, so we need to see what effect this will have on the image. The complete failure to show a particular detail will only occur if the feature is smaller than the apparent focus. There will however be an effect on all detail within the object and on the image.

The effect of the line focus on the image is that the X-rays originating from each side of the focus pass the edges of the object and hit two separate parts of the film creating two images (there are in fact multiple images because X-rays are produced all along the length of the actual focus).

This is the cause of blurring (often called unsharpness, a word that appears in many radiographic texts but not in a dictionary) in the image.

As can be seen in Figure 4.5 positioning the film further away from the object (position b; that is, increasing OFD) will increase the amount of blurring present. The amount of blurring seen with the film in position (a) would not be visible to the naked eye, but that seen with the film in position (b) would start to reduce the level of fine detail observable on the image.

This fact causes some people to mistrust the extended cone paralleling technique for intra-oral radiography. This is because when it is performed correctly the film will be some distance from the object. This fact seems to be completely against the principles discussed so far in this chapter.

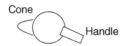

Figure 4.6 Old closed cone X-ray unit

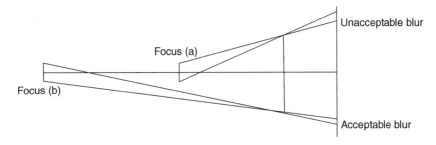

Figure 4.7 Comparison of image blurring at different focus-to-skin distances

PRINCIPLES OF IMAGE FORMATION

The distance between the film/sensor and the object in the paralleling technique does not produce an unacceptable level of blurring because modern X-ray equipment is constructed to compensate for it and reduces blurring to a level not observable on the image. This reduction in blurring is achieved by moving the X-ray tube back from the patient (FFD and FOD are increased).

The X-ray tube head in a dental X-ray unit used to look similar to that in (Figure 4.6).

When the X-ray unit looked like this, the focus (the origin of the X-rays) was just 10 cm from the patients' skin surface. At the time this was not a problem as intra-oral radiography was carried out with the film in close contact with the teeth. Employing film holders (paralleling technique) with this type of X-ray unit would produce the situation given with the film in position (b) in Figure 4.5; the blurring would be unacceptable.

Modern X-ray equipment does not allow the focus to be placed as close to the skin surface as the older type of equipment; the minimum focus-to-skin distance is now 20 cm with many people using a 30 cm distance – hence the name extended cone paralleling. It is the extended cone that maintains the correct distance from the X-ray origin (focus) to the patients' skin surface.

In Figure 4.7 the focus at position (a) shows the effect of using the paralleling technique film/sensor position with an old dental X-ray unit, the focus-to-object distance being 10 cm. Following the path of X-rays from each edge of the focus past one edge of the object shows that they hit the film/sensor at two widely spaced points. The level of blur would be visible to the naked eye and would affect the amount of fine detail visualised on the image.

With the focus at position (b) as it would be with the extended cone paralleling technique, tracing the path of X-rays from each edge of the focus past one edge of the object, as we did for a focus at position (a), shows the two points of the image much closer together.

This would produce a level of blurring not visible to the naked eye, therefore not affecting the fine detail demonstrated.

Of all of the factors needed to produce a good radiographic image, possibly the most important is keeping the object and the film/sensor parallel to each other; if you can achieve this, most of the potential image distortion that could occur will be eliminated.

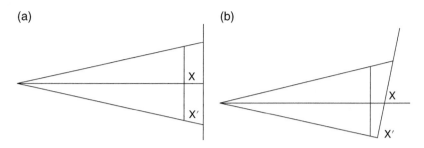

Figure 4.8 (a) Image with film and tooth parallel. (b) Image with film and tooth not parallel

Even some of the mistakes that can be made in positioning the X-ray tube will have a much smaller effect on the final image than would be the case if the film and object were not parallel to each other.

As soon as the parallel relationship between the film/sensor and the object is lost, there will be image distortion no matter how careful or how good you are at performing dental radiography. Image distortion is unavoidable unless the object and image recorder are parallel.

EFFECT OF NONPARALLEL RELATIONSHIP

These two diagrams (Figure 4.8) show a simplified idea of the relative position between the tooth and film with paralleling technique (a) and bisecting angle technique (b). In (b) the film or sensor is held in direct contact with the tooth, and it will be in contact with the crown but will be some distance from the apex because it is held away by the bone and soft tissue of the maxilla or mandible.

Even on this simple diagram it can be clearly seen that in diagram (a) the two parts of the image x and x′ are the same size (as they are in the original object.) In diagram (b) it is clear that x is bigger than x′ a correct 'bisecting' angle would reduce not eliminate the effect.

There has been some image distortion (elongation of the root).

Making sure the geometry is correct is very important for accurate diagnosis.

DIFFERENTIAL ABSORPTION

When we looked at X-ray interactions with matter, we discussed a number of factors that will have an effect on the attenuation of a beam of X-rays. Factors such as atomic number, thickness of material and density are also the factors that produce our radiographic image.

As the beam passes through our patient, it will go through tissues of different atomic number (although there is little variation in soft tissues), different thickness and different density, and the beam energy will also alter the behaviour of the beam and will have an effect on the image.

If we draw a cross-sectional representation of a tooth showing the pulp cavity, dentine and enamel, we can show the effect of each on the number of X-ray quanta that pass through (Figure 4.9).

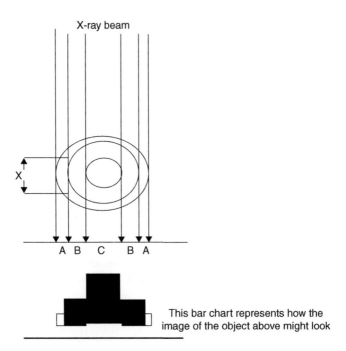

Figure 4.9 Image formation (differential absorption)

In the two areas marked (A) the X-ray quanta have passed through a long column of enamel (X); the enamel is a very dense material, and this long column will absorb quite large number of the quanta so few hit the film or sensor and a white image is produced.

The areas marked (B) show X-ray quanta that have passed through the dentine and here there will be an intermediate amount of absorption.

In (C) the beam, although passing through some enamel and dentine, only passes through relatively thin plates of these materials, and it also passes through the pulp cavity; this will absorb very few quanta. The area of the film or sensor in the middle will be hit by many more X-ray quanta, and a dark area will be produced on the image.

It is worth making an important comparison with photography at this point as it is something that has led to some confusion in the past.

If you overexpose a standard photograph, the image becomes lighter which can lead to white flared areas.

With X-ray images the effect is opposite – the greater the exposure received, the darker the image gets. If an image is grossly overexposed (or over developed), it could become totally black with no diagnostic information.

We have already seen how the tissue factors (atomic number, thickness and density) will affect the image, and we also need to consider how the exposure factors will affect what we see.

The two main factors of exposure to consider are tube current (mA) and the kV. Tube current or mA is what we have been calling filament electrons. We did this to make a clear distinction between them and the electrons in the target material.

Diagrammatic representation of this is probably easier to understand than a long explanation

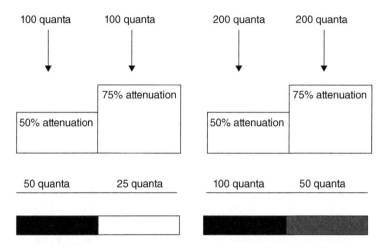

Figure 4.10 Image formation (effect of mA on contrast)

Increasing the tube current will increase the number of X-ray quanta produced in the X-ray tube and passing through the object. This increase in the number of X-rays will increase the overall density of the image (it will get darker). This has to occur because the tissues that the beam passes through will always remove the same percentage of the beam that comes into contact with it.

We learned this when looking at the factors affecting attenuation.

For example, if 100 quanta hit a particular object and it removes 50%, then 50 quanta will hit the film or sensor and produced a particular amount of density (blackness).

If 200 quanta hit the same object, these will again remove 50%, but this means that 100 will now hit the film or sensor producing twice as much density.

In addition to considering the effect of mA on overall density, we have to think about the contrast. Contrast is the difference in density between adjacent areas (or how well do different areas stand out from each other). So, for example, when considering two areas like pulp cavity and dentine, is there just a small difference in density so they do not really stand out from each other (low contrast), or is the density difference large so they are very clearly defined from each other (high contrast)?

The change in contrast will depend on how big the increase in tube current is. Within certain limits increasing the mA will produce an image with better contrast. However further increases in mA may reduce the contrast which will in turn reduce the diagnostic qualities of the image.

A diagrammatic representation of this is probably easier to understand than a long explanation.

In the example shown in Figure 4.10, the materials are two sets of identical attenuators. The only factor that changes is the number of X-ray quanta hitting them and subsequently passing through. When 100 quanta are incident on the blocks, they let through 50 and 25, respectively; the difference in radiographic density (blackness) is the difference that 25 quanta would make.

When 200 quanta are incident on the blocks, they let through 100 and 50, respectively, so the density difference between the two is produced by 50 quanta. The density difference

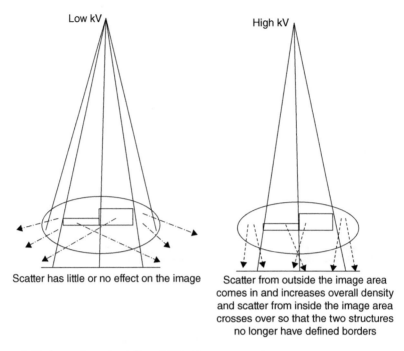

Scatter has little or no effect on the image

Scatter from outside the image area comes in and increases overall density and scatter from inside the image area crosses over so that the two structures no longer have defined borders

Figure 4.11 Image formation (effect of kV on image contrast)

between the two blocks will be twice as big when 200 quanta are incident on the blocks; they will therefore stand out much more clearly from each other. Imagine if this were a small area of caries shown against enamel. Until over exposure is reached.

If the mA is increased further, it will have a negative effect on the contrast. We have shown that at 100 quanta the 50% attenuation block shows black on the image. Any increase in the number of quanta hitting this area cannot make it any darker than black, so it stays as it is. The 75% attenuation block however is not black and can become darker, so as the mA is increased, it effectively catches up the 50% block in terms of how black it looks and the contrast (difference in density) is reduced or even completely disappears (figure 4.10).

So up to the point where any structure reaches maximum density (blackness), any increases in mA will improve contrast; beyond this point further increases in mA will reduce contrast as all other areas will 'catch up' the area that became black first.

This is when the image would reach the point at which we would call it overexposed.

Will kV have a similar effect on the density and contrast of the image?

When discussing the production of X-rays, we saw that the total number of quanta produced is proportional to kV^2. So as kV increases there is potentially a large increase in the number of X-ray quanta that will be directed towards our subject.

This will theoretically have exactly the same effect on density and contrast as increasing the mA (an increase in contrast up to the point where over exposure starts and from that point a reduction in contrast up to the point where there are no density difference, no contrast and no diagnostic information).

There is however a further factor to be taken into account when increasing the kV.

This is the behaviour of any scattered radiation produced within the subject. When in Chapter 3 we described attenuation and the factors affecting it, we saw that attenuation is reduced when a high kV is employed because the scatter is in a more forward direction. It will still hit any detector placed in the path of the main beam.

This is exactly what happens when a high kV beam is directed at a patient – the forward travelling scatter hits the image recording medium, and the effect can be that contrast and sharpness of the image are reduced (Figure 4.11).

The wide-angle scatter at low kV (— · — · — · — ▶) is more likely (though not certain) to miss the film, so it doesn't alter the image of the two structures within the large oval. At high kV the narrow-angle scatter (- - - - - - - - -▶) is more likely to hit the film. The different densities on the image will not only be created by differential absorption in the area of interest but also by scatter coming from outside of the area of interest. This over-all increase in density will reduce the contrast of the image (something like looking at it through frosted glass or a grey screen).

The sharpness is also reduced because scatter produced at the edge of the object can cause additional images of that particular point. The scattered photons move from their original path and hit the image recorder at a slightly different point to where it would have had it not been scattered producing multiple spreading images of that point.

Exposure time will also have an effect on the image – a longer exposure time will cause more quanta to hit the patient and in turn the film or sensor. This will increase the density of the film, and just as with mA there may be an initial increase in contrast, there will be a point where the film becomes overexposed and contrast is reduced.

Longer exposure times also increase the chances that the patient will move during the exposure with a total loss of diagnostic capability in the image.

All of the factors discussed in the formation of the image, imaging geometry and differential absorption, the effects of mA and kV remain the same whatever the image recording system. Remember that what people call digital radiography is simply the use of a digital image recording systems. The X-ray quanta are the same and the way they pass through the patient, or not, are the same. The only factor that changes in a digital system is the way that the image is recorded.

Chapter 5

Imaging with dental X-ray film

Standard film is still a popular recording medium for dental radiographic images as many of its properties are ideal; more and more practices however are changing to digital recording systems.

The construction of the film and its packaging is still a part of most courses covering any aspect of dental radiography. Although the detail is already part of the knowledge base of most dental nurses, it must be included here to complete the text.

DENTAL X-RAY FILM

The film pack has four components (Figure 5.1):

1. Outer plastic cover
   This provides a waterproof, lightproof casing. The outside generally has one plain white face and one that is two-tone. The plain white side is the one that faces the X-ray tube during the X-ray exposure. The inside of the cover is coloured black so that if there were a small pin hole in it the light entering would be absorbed by the black coat.
2. Double fold of black card
   This card has two functions:

   a) It adds physical strength to the film pack to make it less likely that the film bends when in the patients' mouth. This is essential because if the film bends it causes severe distortion of the image.
   b) It also gives additional protection against any light that may leak in through small pin holes in the film cover. As with the black coating inside the cover, the black card will absorb any light passing through and prevent pre-fogging of the image which would reduce the contrast.

3. Film
   Detail of the structure and characteristics of film will be given immediately following this brief description of the film pack.
4. Lead foil
   The first important point to note is that the function of this foil is not the often quoted reduction of radiation dose to the patient. Its function (Figure 5.2) is to preserve the

Basic Guide to Dental Radiography, First Edition. Tim Reynolds.
© 2016 John Wiley & Sons, Ltd. Published 2016 by John Wiley & Sons, Ltd.

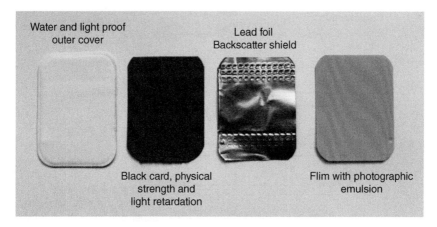

Water and light proof outer cover

Lead foil Backscatter shield

Black card, physical strength and light retardation

Flim with photographic emulsion

Figure 5.1 Components of the dental film pack

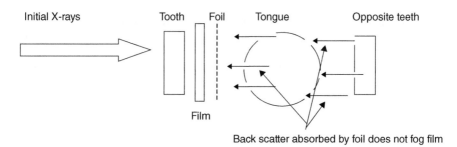

Initial X-rays   Tooth   Foil   Tongue   Opposite teeth

Film

Back scatter absorbed by foil does not fog film

Figure 5.2 Function of the film pack lead foil

image by absorbing X-rays scattered back towards the film from the tongue and other structures at the far side of or back of the mouth. This backscatter could cause fogging of the film (unwanted density) and ghost images of the structures that produced the back scatter. These ghost images could hide important diagnostic information.

THE CONSTRUCTION OF DENTAL FILM

The film base is usually polyester, a material that has many qualities that we need in the base layer of an X-ray film (Figure 5.3). Polyester

Will not change size and shape (it has dimensional stability)
Is very clear and will not reduce image clarity
Is waterproof
Is not flammable
Is flexible so it will pass through automatic processors
Does not react with processing chemicals

The subbing layer is simply there to stick the active (emulsion) layer to the base.

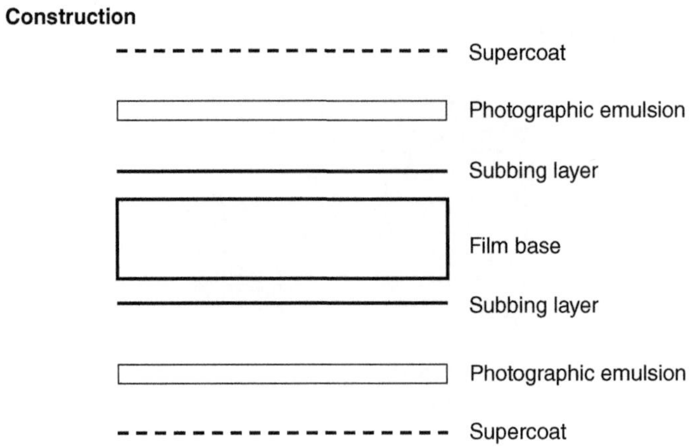

Construction

- - - - - - - - - - - - - - - - - Supercoat

━━━━━━━━━━━━━━━━━━━ Photographic emulsion

━━━━━━━━━━━━━━━━━━━ Subbing layer

━━━━━━━━━━━━━━━━━━━ Film base

━━━━━━━━━━━━━━━━━━━ Subbing layer

━━━━━━━━━━━━━━━━━━━ Photographic emulsion

- - - - - - - - - - - - - - - - - Supercoat

Figure 5.3 Construction of dental X-ray film

The emulsion is the active imaging substance, and it is where the X-ray quanta react with the film to form the picture that we use to make the diagnosis. It consists of gelatine and the active ingredients called silver halides.

The supercoat is a layer of hardened gelatine that protects the surface of the image from physical harm.

FILM EMULSION

The active emulsion is gelatine and a silver halide (this means a compound of silver that reacts to light and X-rays). Two common halides are silver iodide and silver bromide. In dental X-ray film the halide is silver bromide, and its chemical formula is AgBr (Ag being silver and Br bromine). The molecules of silver bromide are held in a crystal structure suspended in gelatine with each crystal containing many of the active molecules.

Remember, in Chapter 1, when we discussed elements, compounds, atoms and molecule. We said that the outer electron shells of atoms govern their chemical properties and make the chemical bonds that cause the atoms of elements to join together in making the molecules of compounds.

In Chapter 3 when discussing the details of X-ray interactions with matter, we said that once an atom has been ionised (has an electron ejected), its chemical properties are changed. This makes a difference to the elements that the atom will and will not bond with.

These two facts coupled with differential absorption give us all the information we need to understand how the image is made on a film emulsion.

When a silver bromide molecule interacts with a quantum of X-rays (Figure 5.4) and is ionised, the two components drift apart because removing the electron through ionisation weakens the chemical bond between them.

After the X-ray quantum has ionised the silver bromide, the molecule separates. Note that the silver has a positive charge sign. The number of AgBr molecules separating will be proportional to the number of quanta interacting with the crystals of the active emulsion (Figure 5.5). This will of course depend on the materials (tissues) that the beam passes through.

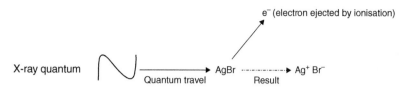

Figure 5.4 Silver bromide reaction to X-ray exposure

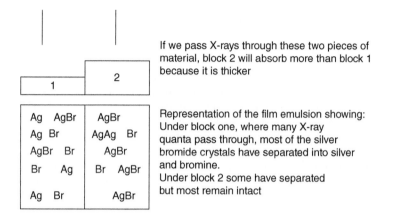

If we pass X-rays through these two pieces of material, block 2 will absorb more than block 1 because it is thicker

Representation of the film emulsion showing:
Under block one, where many X-ray quanta pass through, most of the silver bromide crystals have separated into silver and bromine.
Under block 2 some have separated but most remain intact

Figure 5.5 Effects on the film emulsion of different levels of radiation exposure

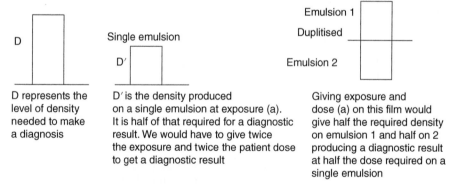

D represents the level of density needed to make a diagnosis

D′ is the density produced on a single emulsion at exposure (a). It is half of that required for a diagnostic result. We would have to give twice the exposure and twice the patient dose to get a diagnostic result

Giving exposure and dose (a) on this film would give half the required density on emulsion 1 and half on 2 producing a diagnostic result at half the dose required on a single emulsion

Figure 5.6 Effect of duplitising the emulsion

The positive charge on the silver atom plays an important part in the later development of the image during processing.

When this film is processed, the area that lay under block one will come out dark grey or black (it will have high radiographic density) and the area under block 2 will be light grey or nearly clear (low radiographic density). The image will remain invisible (latent image) until the film is developed.

An important detail of film construction to note is the fact that there is active emulsion on both sides of the base, and the film is said to be duplitised. This arrangement allows us to produce our diagnostic image at just half of the dose that would be required if there were only one active layer of emulsion (Figure 5.6).

IMAGING WITH DENTAL X-RAY FILM

FILM CHARACTERISTICS

The way in which a film responds when exposed to X-rays is defined by its characteristic curve. This is a graph of its response to different levels of exposure. The curve will tell us how fast a film is (i.e. how much exposure is required to reach a certain level of radiographic density) and also tells us how much contrast there will be (how much change in density will there be with small changes in level of exposure) (Figure 5.7).

Characteristic curve of a film

Key points on the characteristic curve

D_{fog}: This is a level of density that exists on a film even if no X-ray exposure is made. It is there because of colour dyes added to the base to prevent dazzle.

Toe: This is the point at which the film starts to react in a useful way to X-ray exposure. Below this level increases in exposure have very little effect on the density produced, no useful diagnostic information would be recorded. This is because changes in the density would be too small to be detected by the human eye.

Straight-line portion: This is the main diagnostic section of the film, here changes to exposure here will cause significant changes in the density of the film. So the difference in attenuation between the healthy enamel and an area of caries will produce large density differences on the film, and diagnostic information is clear.

Shoulder: This is the point at which the film approaches its maximum density and response to further exposure is reduced. Here the difference in attenuation between the healthy enamel and an area of caries would not produce enough density difference to make the diagnosis. This would be the area of overexposure discussed in Chapter 4.

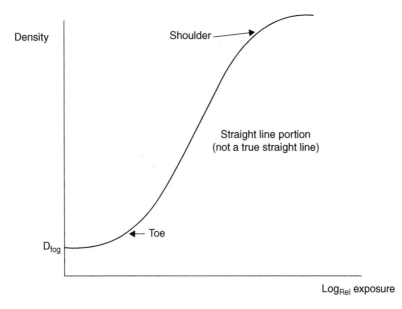

Figure 5.7 Film characteristic curve features

The fact the exposure axis is labelled $\log_{rel}$ exposure is not important; it's a mathematical trick to reduce the length of the axis to make the graph more manageable. For our purposes we can just think of that axis as exposure pure and simple.

FILM SPEED

Film speed as previously stated is an expression for how much density will be produced on a film for a given level of exposure. Faster film allows us to reduce the dose to the patient but still produce enough density to make a diagnosis from the image. Over the past few years the general advice has been to move from the use of D speed dental X-ray film to E or E/F in order to make a general reduction to the radiation doses delivered to patients.

The speed of a film is indicated by its general position on the graph of its characteristics (Figure 5.8). The further to the left of the axis that a curve appears, the greater the film response to exposure will be.

Looking at the two characteristic curves in Figure 5.8, we see that Film A reaches the required density at a much lower level of exposure than Film B. Film A is therefore the faster of the two films.

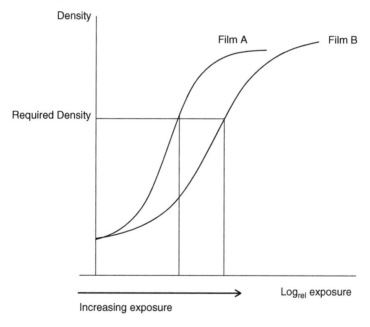

Figure 5.8 Characteristic curve position and film speed

FILM CONTRAST

The contrast characteristics of the film are determined by the slope of the 'straight-line' section of the curve, and this slope is called the gamma of the curve. Sometimes instead of looking at only the central straight-line portion, the average gradient across the whole

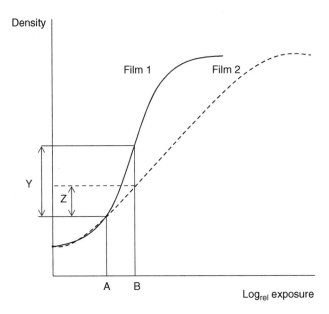

Figure 5.9 Characteristic curve shape and film contrast

curve is used. It doesn't matter in particular which type of reading is used as long as we remember that the slope will tell us how much contrast we will see on the image.

For a film to provide good contrast (i.e. a wide range of densities from very dark to very light), we need it to produce a big density difference when there is very little difference in exposure to the film.

Film contrast characteristics

In the example given here there are two points labelled A and B. These represent different levels of exposure reaching the film: A may be the X-rays that come through the dentine and B the X-rays that come through the pulp cavity (Figure 5.9).

To see which film gives the best contrast, we just need to draw a vertical line from points A and B up to the characteristic curve of each film. Where the vertical lines hit the characteristic curve, we then take a horizontal line across the density axis of the graph. The film that produces two points on the density axis that are further apart is the film with the best contrast characteristics.

Film 2 (the dotted characteristic curve) produces two points that are distance apart (Z), and Film 1 (solid curve) gives us two points that are much further apart (Y).

This shows that Film 1 will produce a much bigger density difference between the pulp cavity and the dentine; it will give images of much higher contrast.

FILM LATITUDE

One disadvantage of high-contrast film is that you have to be much more accurate with the setting of your exposure factors because as contrast characteristics increase film latitude decreases. Latitude can be described as the degree by which you can over- or underexpose an image and still get a diagnostic result.

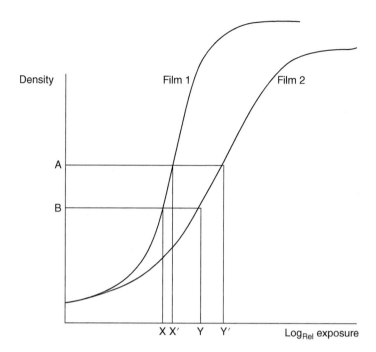

Figure 5.10 Characteristic curve effects on film and exposure latitude

Film (latitude) characteristics

If we say that for an image to be of any diagnostic value, the density must be between points A and B. We see that Film 1 only allows a narrow range of exposures X to X', but Film 2 allows a much wider range Y to Y'. So the range of exposure allowable in producing a diagnostic image is greater on Film 2. Film 2 has the greater latitude (Figure 5.10).

There are two terms related to this last fact, film latitude and exposure latitude. Film latitude describes the full extent of exposures the film can be subjected to in order to give densities that fall in the useful area between the toe and shoulder of the curve.

Exposure latitude describes the full range of exposures that would produce a diagnostic result for any particular examination.

It is not true that faster films necessarily have lower contrast characteristics as it is possible to create fast film and a slower one with the same or very similar gradients.

CONTRAST AND SPEED

In the example given here it is easy to see that Film 1 will reach any given density at a lower exposure value than Film 2. Film 1 is therefore a faster film than Film 2.

If however we look at the contrast characteristics (Figure 5.11) by selecting a range of densities A to B and look at the exposure spread needed to produce this density difference, we see that on Film 1 the exposure spread is X' to X and on Film 2 the spread is Y' to Y, in each case the spread being exactly the same. The films will therefore produce

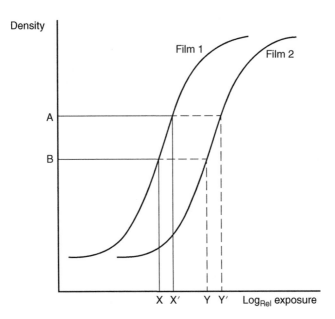

Figure 5.11 Independence of speed and contrast characteristics

exactly the same density difference between the pulp cavity and dentine, but Film 1 will do it at a lower exposure and lower patient dose.

The thought, often quoted, that modern fast films produce low-contrast images is not necessarily true, and it is just as likely, if not more, so that the low contrast is caused by the higher average kV produced by the constant potential or ripple voltage forms of modern X-ray equipment.

FILM PROCESSING

Many times you will hear film processing referred to as developing but that is only one part of the process.

The film goes through five stages: development, rinse, fixing, washing and drying. If this process is carried out properly in a manual (often called dip) tank, it takes approximately 1 h.

DEVELOPER

Immediately following the X-ray exposure the film holds a latent image, and all of the information is there, in the form of ionised and separated silver and bromine atoms within the crystals of the emulsion, but it is invisible.

The purpose of the developer is to make this latent image visible. It does this by increasing the concentration of separated metallic silver atoms. Metallic silver is naturally black in colour.

IMAGING WITH DENTAL X-RAY FILM

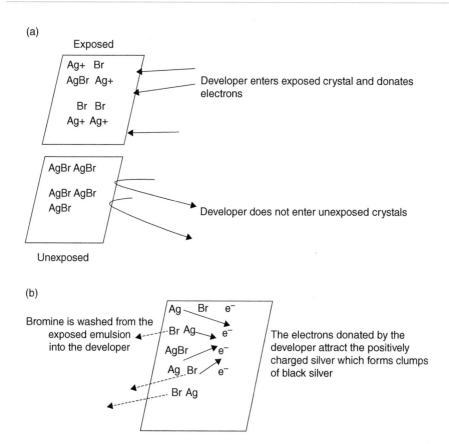

Figure 5.12 (a) Action of developer on exposed and unexposed crystals. (b) Developer action; electrons attracting positive silver ions in the emulsion

The developer needs to be both quick acting and selective. By selective we mean that it develops (collects silver atoms) only in those crystals that have been exposed to X-rays. Speed of action and high selectivity are mutually exclusive (if you have one you don't have the other). Developing agents usually consist of a combination of agents so that the desired characteristics of speed and selectivity can be produced in the correct balance. There are many other chemicals in developing solution, and they perform functions such as the following: preserve the alkalinity, activate the constituents, harden the emulsion and prevent excessive fogging (unwanted density) on the film.

The developer is a particular type of chemical substance called a reducing agent, and all that we need to understand about this type of agent is that it donates electrons to other substances. In donating electrons the developer itself becomes oxidised. You may have heard the term oxidised applied to the developer that has become old and useless, and many people mistakenly believe this to mean it has taken in lots of oxygen rather than it being the description of a chemical reaction. Oxidation in this case is the depletion of its supply of electrons.

There are a number of different theories as to exactly how developer works. That shown in Figure 5.12 is one of the ones that has been widely accepted.

The unexposed crystals in the emulsion have a structure that does not allow the developer to penetrate and donate electrons. However if the developing solution is, too strong, too hot or the film is left in for too long unexposed crystals will start to develop and turn black.

Exposing the crystal to X-rays (light would do the same) produces a weakness in the crystal, and this weakness allows the developer to penetrate and to donate electrons. The donated electrons with their negative charge attract the positively charged silver atoms.

From the previous chapters we know that as more X-rays fall upon the film, more silver atoms are released from the silver bromide molecules through ionisation. As the concentration of silver atoms increases, the image becomes blacker in that particular area because the silver atoms clump together following development.

The developer, put simply, gathers the free silver atoms in each of the crystals into clumps.

If there has been little exposure, there are few free silver atoms and the image in that area will be clear to pale grey.

If there is an intermediate level of exposure, the image is light to mid-grey.

Where there is heavy exposure, dark grey to black areas appear on the film.

The free bromine is washed out of the emulsion into the developer solution. This is why the old developer is brown in colour. NB: This is not the cause of the brown staining seen on some old films when they are taken from the store.

The old developer becomes less able to develop the film for two reasons: it has fewer electrons to donate to the exposed crystals, and the bromine acts as a chemical suppressor to the developer action.

At the end of the developer cycle as much developer as possible must be removed from the emulsion. In manual tanks this is done by a spray rinse, and in an automatic processor the film passes through a pair of rollers like an old-fashioned clothes mangle (they squeeze the developer off the film).

Developing faults

Over-development

This could occur because the developer is too hot, the concentration is too high (too strong), or the film is in the developer for too long.

The developer being too strong is unlikely to happen with modern premixed developers, and similarly the film being in the developer for too long is unlikely to happen in an automatic processor unless it sticks while passing through the developer rollers, and it does however happen in manual tanks.

The result of over-development is a high density image, and in extreme circumstances even unexposed crystals will start to develop and turn grey or black. The overall effect on the image is a reduction in contrast. The areas that should be black is still black, but all the other areas increase in density so that all areas are closer to the same density.

Under-development

This could be due to low developer temperature, exhausted developer or the film not being in developer long enough.

The film not being in developer long enough can only happen in automatic processors that do not have low fluid level warning lights (Figure 5.13).

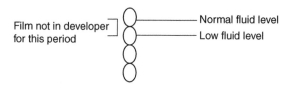

Figure 5.13 Developing time and effect of low developer levels

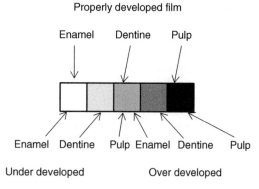

Figure 5.14 Effect of development on film density and contrast

The effect of under-development is a generally reduced density in the film. There may not be sufficient density to diagnose problems round the apex or bony margins.

Contrast will be also reduced because the usually dark structures become lighter and the light areas are closer to the density they would have on a properly developed film. This means the densities of all structures become more nearly equal and lie towards the lighter end of the density scale, contrast between them is reduced (Figure 5.14). Over development has a similar effect but all structures would have increased density.

Water splashes

If water is splashed onto the film prior to development, it makes the emulsion damp. When the film passes into the developer, the chemicals are allowed to pass into the emulsion more easily in those damp parts, and they will be over-developed. Water splashes will show as small dark areas and, unless they are recognised, could be thought to be pathological changes.

Air bells

This is a problem exclusive to manual processing. When the film is placed into the developer, it should be agitated (shaken around) to remove air bubbles from its surface. If the air bubbles remain, they prevent the developer from contacting and interacting with the film, and multiple small under-developed areas will be seen on the final image.

After the development cycle is finished, the developer is removed from the film and the film passes into the fixer.

FIXER

This part of the processing cycle has two functions: it makes the image permanent and it hardens the emulsion.

Fixing agents contain ammonium thiosulphate as their main active ingredient (it is not important that you remember this, but it will explain a fixer fault that is often attributed to developer); it also accounts for the smell if you leave the lid off the processor particularly in warm weather.

Like developing solution they contains other chemicals that maintain the acidity, harden the emulsion and prevent the fixer from deteriorating too quickly.

The fixer hardens the emulsion to prevent mechanical damage such as scratches, which would reduce the diagnostic quality of the film.

The fixer makes the image permanent by ensuring that any additional exposure to X-rays, light or other stimulating influence will not add to the density of the image (i.e. no further exposure of the emulsion can take place).

During fixing all of the unexposed crystals remaining in the emulsion are washed off into the fixer solution. Once these unexposed crystals are removed, the image can be exposed to unlimited X-rays or light, and no additional density will be produced on the image (Figure 5.15).

Here we see two crystals in the emulsion, one exposed and developed and the other completely unexposed. They are surrounded by fixer that has no effect on the exposed, developed, crystal, but it does remove all of the unexposed silver bromide (AgBr) crystals. At the end of the process the unexposed crystal will be completely clear and has no active (exposable) silver bromide molecules within it.

Fixer faults

Over-fixing

It is not really possible to over-fix a film as its aim is to remove all unexposed crystals and it will not do more than this. Theoretically it would be possible if the film were left for a prolonged period for the emulsion to start to lift from the film base; this however for all practical purposes can be ignored.

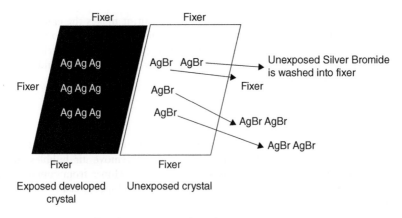

Figure 5.15 Function of the fixer on exposed emulsions

Under-fixing

As with under-developing under-fixing can be caused by low temperature, insufficient time or exhaustion of the fixer.

The two common results of fixer problems are as follows:

1. The film exits the automatic processor damp. This is because the first of the fixer functions to fail in adverse conditions is the hardening of the emulsion. When the hardener does not function properly, the emulsion remains soft and it takes in too much water. The excess water makes it impossible for the emulsion to dry in the time allowed in an automatic processor.
2. The film will have a green tint after processing, and this is because the unexposed crystals remain on the emulsion (parts of the image will look similar to the appearance of a film taken straight out of the box). The film is said to have a milky green opalescence.

WASHING

This is the final wet stage of the processing cycle, and its function is to remove all remaining chemicals from the emulsion to the image archival permanence (making sure it doesn't deteriorate during storage).

In manual or automatic processing it is important that there is constant water flow so that the film is always surrounded by fresh clean water. If this is not achieved, the chemicals (fixer) washed off into the water simply come into contact with the film again and are deposited on the surface, the film coming out of the processor still covered in fixer instead of being clean.

Washing faults insufficient washing

If there is inadequate washing there will be a fixer in the emulsion. During storage, this fixer starts to decompose, and sulphur products are separated from other constituents. This sulphur gives the image a yellow brown tint, and it will smell sharp and pungent a bit like rotten eggs.

So brown staining on the image is not due to old brown developer but to residual fixer that was not washed off the emulsion and has decomposed during storage.

DRYING THE FILM

Drying is the final stage of processing, and we need the film to be completely dry before handling because the emulsion hardeners in the developer and fixer are not completely effective until the film is dry. Handling a wet or damp film will very easily produce scratches in the emulsion or fingermark imprints that may affect later diagnostic capability.

Manual processing

Manual processing taking the time from dry to dry is a long one (when it is performed correctly).

Developing: In order for the slower more selective agent in the developer to work, this part of the cycle will be in the region for 5 min.

Spray rinse: Approximately 20 seconds.

Fixer: Usually double the developing time for 10 min; the film will look clear after 5 min, but for the fixer to work completely, the full 10 min is required.

Washing: 20 min in constantly flowing and changing water is required to remove all of the residual fixer from the emulsion.

Drying: This will depend on temperature and airflow, but on average the time taken to completely dry the emulsion will be 20–30 min.

Dry-to-dry time in a set of manual tanks is therefore around 1 h, so you can see why some alternative was necessary.

Automatic processors: These are much quicker than this because in general higher concentrations of more active chemicals are used than was the case when only manual systems were available. The average temperature is also higher, and this speeds up any chemical reaction including the development and fixing of photographic emulsions.

IMAGING WITH DENTAL X-RAY FILM

Chapter 6

Digital imaging recording

It is important to note that this chapter is titled 'Digital image recording' and not digital radiography.

This is quite deliberate as the second term (digital radiography or digital X-rays) has led some to believe that the actual X-rays are in some way different from those used when employing standard dental film as the recording system.

This is not the case. To convert from film to digital dental radiography, all you need to do is select the type of recording system you want and cancel your film order, and you can use the same X-ray machine that you have always used.

The radiation is just as dangerous and it is subject to all of the same legally enforceable regulations.

There are three types of digital image recorder that you may come across: phosphor plates, wireless sensors and sensors with wire connections to the computer.

It is not necessary for you to know the exact details of how the electronic circuits work or what phosphor materials are used or indeed the precise details of how they function (this is after all a basic guide). What we will include in this section is a general idea of how these systems work.

Digital radiographs are produced in basically the same way as images on film; the X-ray beam passes through the patient and will be absorbed in different quantities by different tissues. Some parts of the phosphor or sensor receive many X-ray quanta (those passing through the pulp cavity), and some will receive very few (those passing through the enamel). The result will be a series of light and dark areas making up the picture we recognise as the radiograph.

All that is different is the way in which the image is captured and saved to the patient's notes.

TYPES OF DIGITAL IMAGE RECORDER

Phosphor plates

There are many different phosphor plates on the market. In general their dimensions are very similar to the standard dental X-ray film that people are familiar with. Some are slightly more rigid than film and others slightly less so.

Basic Guide to Dental Radiography, First Edition. Tim Reynolds.
© 2016 John Wiley & Sons, Ltd. Published 2016 by John Wiley & Sons, Ltd.

Although there are structural differences between the phosphor plates manufactured by each company, they all work on very similar principles.

The image is stored on the plate just as an image is stored in the emulsion of the film, and just as with film the phosphor plate image is invisible until it is processed.

There are two major differences between film and phosphor plates:

1. The image on film is produced by the ionisation and eventual separation of silver bromide crystals. In the phosphor plate; it is created by a sort of suspended excitation.
2. The image on film is processed through a series of wet processing chemicals; the phosphor plates are processed completely dry with laser light and electronics.

We have seen in earlier chapters that excitation is a transient effect, short lived and producing no permanent change in the atom.

We also said that one of the characteristics of X-rays is the fluoroscopic effect; this means that in some materials the absorption of X-ray energy results in the immediate emission of light. There will be more low-energy light quanta than there were high-energy X-ray quanta; this effect is utilised in the intensifying screens in traditional OPG cassettes to reduce the X-ray dose needed to form an image.

The two effects discussed earlier are related because initial excitation (raising the energy level of electrons) leads to the emission of light as the electrons fall back to their original energy level.

The light output will be equal to the energy given to the electrons in raising them from their starting position. They have to give up this energy because the atom must always return to its lowest energy state, and electrons can only lie in any particular shell if they have the correct level of energy (Chapter 1).

All of the energy absorbed from the X-ray beam must be given up as the atom returns to its natural state.

We see here (Figure 6.1) X-ray quanta passing close to the valence band of an atom. The electrons in that band are excited to a higher energy level, but when the stimulus of the X-ray quanta is removed, the electrons fall immediately back to the valence band. As they fall, they give off light to reduce their energy to the level required for them to exist in their original position.

This is an example of the fluoroscopic effect.

Another characteristic of X-rays is the phenomenon of phosphorescence. It is very similar to the fluoroscopic effect with one major difference; that is, instead of an

DIGITAL IMAGING RECORDING

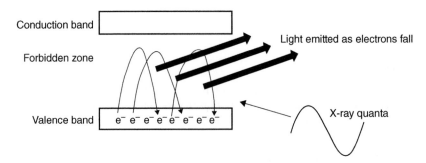

Figure 6.1 Fluorescence (excited electrons fall back into place emitting light)

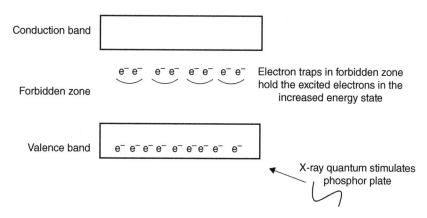

Conduction band

Forbidden zone — e⁻ e⁻ e⁻ e⁻ e⁻ e⁻ e⁻ e⁻   Electron traps in forbidden zone hold the excited electrons in the increased energy state

Valence band — e⁻ e⁻e⁻e⁻ e⁻ e⁻e⁻ e⁻ e⁻

X-ray quantum stimulates phosphor plate

Figure 6.2 Phosphorescence (electrons held at increased energy levels for a time)

immediate return by the electron in its original energy level and immediate emission of light, there is a delayed effect and there will be a time lag between the end of the X-ray stimulus and the emission of light.

With phosphor plate imaging, the material selected for the plate must be capable of holding the electrons in their higher energy state until we are ready for them to be released. This really means they must be held there until we release them (Figure 6.2).

One of the materials of choice for this function is barium fluorobromide.

To enhance the properties we desire, the barium fluorobromide has one of the following additives: europium or caesium bromide.

For a basic understanding of dental radiography, you do not need to remember the names of the materials used, but it is included for those who wish to use this text as additional reading for a more serious level of study.

Barium fluorobromide effectively has electron traps in the forbidden zone between the two outer electron energy bands, that is, the valence band and the conduction band.

The europium or caesium bromide increases the ability of the molecules to hold electrons suspended in their excited state; the way in which they do this is not relevant to a study of this type.

The phosphor material is supported on a polyester base; there is also a reflective layer to maximise the capture of light quanta when the plate is processed through the reader.

The example shown is not an accurate representation of the effect as the excited electrons in the phosphor material are not held in little cups; in fact there is no physical trap, but it is a chemical effect. The cups do however make it easier to understand what is involved in the imaging process.

The image is produced in exactly the same way as an image recorded on film, that is, differential absorption.

If we pass 100 X-ray quanta through the two materials below each having different attenuating power, we will have different numbers of quanta passing through.

The part of phosphor plate that lies under the 50% attenuating material (say dentine) receives many X-ray quanta, and there are many electrons held in traps within the forbidden zone (Figure 6.3).

The part that lies under the 75% attenuator (enamel) will receive few X-ray quanta, and few electrons are held in traps.

If we pass 100 X-ray quants through each of these materials of different attenuating power we will see different numbers of quanta passing through each of them

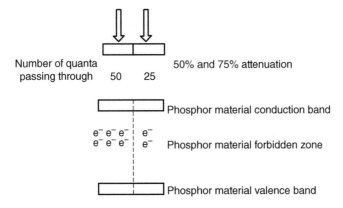

Number of quanta   50% and 75% attenuation
passing through   50   25

Figure 6.3 Image formation in phosphor plates

This is very similar to there being areas where different numbers of silver bromide molecules are broken apart, producing different levels of density.

The image on the phosphor plate will remain invisible; it is simply stored energy until it is processed to form the final image for diagnosis.

The image processors for these plates have a number of different designs, but the process will be similar.

The electrons in the traps must be stimulated sufficiently for them to effectively jump out of the traps. Once they are out of the traps, they follow the usual laws of physics and fall back to their original position (remember atoms must always be in the lowest possible energy state). As they fall they must give up the additional energy they have been holding, and this energy is given up as blue light. The intensity of light given off from each area of the sensor is proportional to the number of X-ray quanta that hit that area and therefore to the number of electrons held in suspension. In the example given more light will be emitted from the area of the plate lying under the 50% attenuator than from under the 75% attenuator.

The plate holding the image is stimulated by laser light; this gives the electrons just enough energy for them to jump from the trapped position and to then fall to their original energy level.

The small amount of light given off is detected by a photomultiplier tube (light intensity-increasing device) and is then converted to a digital electronic signal.

Following the whole sequence through, we have the following:

An area of low attenuation (pulp cavity) allows many X-ray quanta to pass through.
The large number of X-ray quanta hitting the phosphor causes large numbers of electrons to be held in the forbidden zone.
Laser light releases the electrons from their trapped position.
The electrons return to their original energy level.
Light is given off as the excess energy is released.
Light energy is increased by the photomultiplier tubes.
Light is converted to a digital signal and passed to the computer.

DIGITAL IMAGING RECORDING

After the image has been recorded, the phosphor plate has to be subjected to high-intensity light long enough for all of the electrons in traps to be returned to their original energy level. This process completely removes all image information from the plate.

After the image has been completely removed, the plate (unlike film) is ready to use again.

From the previous descriptions, and as previously mentioned, you will see that the images produced on phosphor plates are not visible until the plate has been processed through the reader – much the same as we have to process a film to visualise the image. The difference is that there are no messy processing chemicals and no image quality problems arising from poor processing conditions.

There is a time lag from pressing the exposure button to viewing the image, though this time lag is not as extended as it would be when using film to record the image.

Charge-coupled devices

The charge-coupled device (CCD) is a digital image sensor that allows almost immediate viewing of the image; this is possible because the image is passed from the sensor to the computer screen through a USB connection.

The charge-coupled sensors are somewhat more bulky than the phosphor plate sensors because the electronic components that convert the X-ray quanta image into a digital electronic signal are contained within the sensor itself.

There are two ways in which the X-ray quanta are converted into digital image information:

1. A light-sensitive material detects light produced by a scintillation crystal (this converts X-ray quanta to light); the light is converted to electric charge through a second layer of material acting as a photodiode. (A photodiode creates charge through its exposure to light.)
2. An X-ray-sensitive material converts X-ray quanta into charge, it is effectively the release of electrons through ionisation of the material that creates this charge.

Both of these types of sensors are bulky when compared with film and phosphor plates, but those utilising a scintillation layer may be slightly thicker due to this additional component.

Whichever system produces the charge, the process from this point is similar. The charge is temporarily stored in tiny capacitors (charge-storing device). Once the image acquisition is complete, the stored charge is removed from the capacitors in the form of a small voltage. The voltage is measured and converted into the appropriate digital signal strength (light or dark image point).

Each of the charge-storing devices represents a picture point and each has its own wire connecting it to the computer. There will be at least two million individual picture points called pixels in a standard intra-oral digital sensor.

The explanations given previously are not meant to fully explain the operating principles of CCD; to do so requires a reasonably detailed study of semiconductor and transistor theory.

Many systems now employ complementary metal–oxide–semiconductor (CMOS) technology; this uses a balanced series of semiconductor materials to improve performance; in particular they are low noise (electronic interference) and low static power use.

Imaging sequence through these CCD devices:

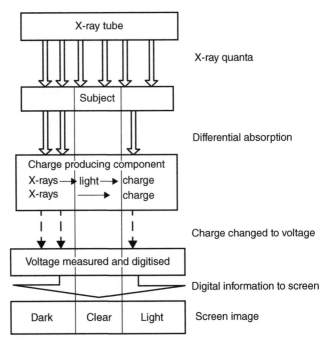

Figure 6.4 Charge-coupled devices (imaging sequence)

The wires that connect these systems to the computer can be limiting in some circumstances, and an alternative technology is to utilise Wi-Fi technology to pass the image from the sensor to the computer. Access to the image in both is immediate.

A simplified summary of the imaging sequence through a CCD (Figure 6.4).

DIGITAL IMAGE RECORDING ADVANTAGES

All of the digital image recording systems described have advantages when compared to analogue (film) images:

Problems arising from the use of processing chemicals are eliminated (image quality and personal safety considerations are reduced).

On-screen images provide an excellent aid to instruction (for students or patients).

There is some potential for the reduction of the patients' dose, and this is not large when a well maintained processor and EF speed film system are compared with a digital system. Typically dose savings of 10–15% may be achieved when comparing good digital with good film systems.

Images can be easily transferred between practitioners when required.

The sharper (enhanced) edges between areas of different density will produce an apparent increase in the detail demonstrated (note this is apparent not actual).

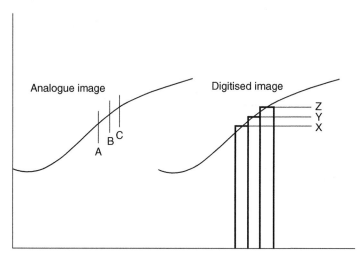

Figure 6.5 Comparison of digital/analogue image

DIGITAL ANALOGUE DETAIL COMPARISON

The previous graph shows an analogue image to the left and the effect of digitising that image on the right. If we take three image points, A, B and C, there will be a gradual transition of density on the analogue image which may be difficult to see (Figure 6.5).

When this image is digitised, the points A, B and C are in the centre of the rectangular columns, and the width of the columns represents a pixel (individual picture point). The difference in density between these pixels is represented by the points X, Y and Z. There are very definite steps in density that are much easier to see than gradual changes in the analogue image.

Digital images can be manipulated after acquisition. There are a number of things that can be done to improve the diagnostic information available:

Colour can be added (different greyscales are allocated a colour).
Images can be embossed (this gives an impression of three-dimensional imaging).
Localisation and magnification of areas.
Callipers can be added for accurate imaging.
The image can be inverted (black to white, white to black).
Density and contrast can be altered.

DIGITAL IMAGE DENSITY MANIPULATION

Increasing the density of the image effectively does the equivalent of moving a films characteristic curve to the left. An area of the patient producing exposure A to the image recording device would give density 1 with the curve in position Y. When the curve is moved to the left (position X), the same exposure A gives much greater density 2 (Figure 6.6).

DIGITAL IMAGING RECORDING

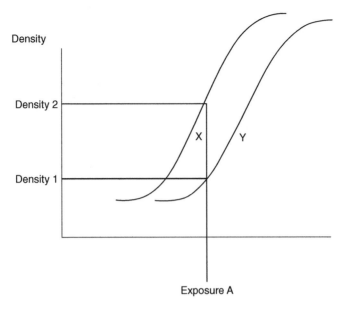

Figure 6.6 Manipulation of density in digital images

The level of density shown is predicted by tracing the line indicating the level of exposure vertically until it hits each of the film curves.

A note of caution when considering this point is that if the image is underexposed, there is insufficient penetration by enough quanta to produce diagnostic information around the apical region. Increasing the density of the image cannot make this information appear. It simply makes the image more aesthetically appealing.

CONTRAST MANIPULATION

Changing the contrast of the image is achieved by electronically altering the slope (gradient) of the curve so that two areas in the patient providing exposures A (photons passing through the enamel) and B (photons passing through the dentine) to the sensor can be made to stand out much more clearly from each other (Figure 6.7).

In the original set parameters, gradient (slope) 1, there will be a small density difference (Y) between the two areas of exposure, and this may be difficult to see. This will be a low-contrast image.

Changing the contrast so that the sensor has gradient (slope) 2 means that these two areas will have a larger density difference (Z) and they will be much more clearly differentiated from each other. This will be a higher-contrast image and different structures will stand out more clearly.

It is also possible to enlarge images on the screen to aid teaching, but this only improves visualisation of structures up to a point. But eventually as the image gets bigger, the image breaks down into visible square blocks (you can see the pixels but not the image). Try this with an image on your mobile phone.

There are many advantages in digital image recording but also some pitfalls.

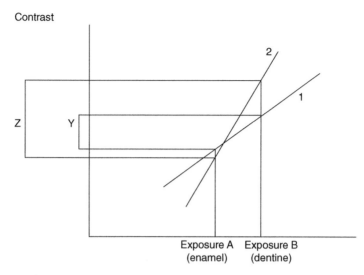

Figure 6.7 Manipulation of contrast in digital imaging

It is possible to put so much effort into image manipulation that the practitioner loses sight of the original aim of producing the image.

There are also many people who still believe that digital radiography is capable of a 90% dose reduction when compared with analogue film images; when comparing the best of both systems, digital gives a best of around 15% reduction in dose.

It is also believed that there is more information on a digital, but because of the way the pixels are formed (see Figure 6.5), there is technically less detail as some parts of the analogue image disappear in the averaging of a group of densities to form the pixel. It is unlikely that the missing information would be available for diagnosis because the human eye would not pick up density changes as subtle as those that were cut out. Film and digital recording systems produce around the same level of resolution (fine detail).

DIGITAL IMAGING RECORDING

Chapter 7

X-ray equipment

INTRA-ORAL

Intra-oral dental X-ray equipment needs to be light and easily manoeuvrable close to the patient's face so that the correct positioning can be achieved.

It also needs to be safe; there is after all a minimum of 60 000 V just 20 cm from the patient's face, and then there is the radiation.

In large items of X-ray equipment in hospitals, there used to be a large high-tension (step-up) transformer in the corner of the room with cables of up to 1 inch diameter from the transformer to the X-ray tube head. The transformer was full of mineral oil and so was the X-ray tube head; the units were therefore referred to as twin tank units.

Similar cables would have severely reduced the manoeuvrability of a dental X-ray tube, so they were constructed as single tank units, and this means that all of the components to generate the operating kVp and those supplying the filament are contained within the tube housing (Figure 7.1).

For a number of years now, even large X-ray machines in hospitals are constructed on the same principle.

DENTAL INTRA-ORAL TUBE HEAD

Tube exit port detail

In the diagram shown Figure 7.2 the solid arrows show the part of the X-ray beam that will pass through the exit port to eventually hit the patient and form the image. The arrows with the broken lines come from the X-ray tube at a much wider angle and hit the internal lead collimator and are not allowed to exit the tube housing.

The external collimator ensures that the beam does not extend beyond the required limits.

Basic Guide to Dental Radiography, First Edition. Tim Reynolds.
© 2016 John Wiley & Sons, Ltd. Published 2016 by John Wiley & Sons, Ltd.

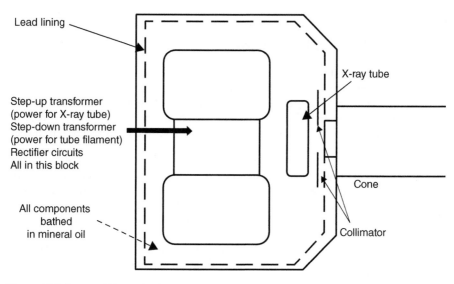

Figure 7.1 Intra-oral X-ray tube housing

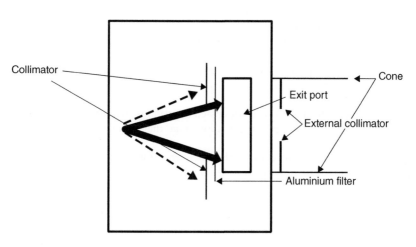

Figure 7.2 X-ray tube exit port detail

Many standard X-ray machines are fitted with round collimators but can be adapted to rectangular with the fitting of an integrated rectangular collimator/cone or a universal rectangular attachment.

This detail also shows the aluminium filter that must be placed in the path of the beam; remember this is an illustration and not all X-ray equipment will have these features placed in exactly these positions, (the filter may be outside the port), however all of the features will be present in all equipment. In some cases the collimator may be an integral part of the cone rather than being situated within the tube housing.

Mineral oil

The oil in the tube housing has two functions:

1. It provides electrical insulation so that the 60–70 kV potential across the X-ray tube cannot make the tube housing electrically live.
2. When heat from the target reaches the glass envelope of the tube through radiation of heat from the target and through conduction by the anode block, convection currents in the oil carry it from the glass envelope to the casing where it is removed to the air.

The lead lining prevents radiation from leaving the tube housing other than through the small exit port. This provides radiation safety for the patient because it allows the X-rays to pass only towards the examination area. The lead lining also protects any members of staff or other persons that are required to be in the general area.

The cone fitted over the exit port of the X-ray tube housing has two functions:

1. It provides a visual guide to the full extent of the spread of the X-ray beam. An open-ended cone is now a legal requirement on dental X-ray machines so that people are aware of the spread of the beam. The old-style pointed cones that gave a false impression of the beam being narrowly focussed towards the teeth should have been removed from use.
2. The cone also maintains the correct focus-to-skin distance; the current minimum focus-to-skin distance is 20 cm. Previously 10 cm was allowed when using 50 kV X-ray machines, but these should not have been used since the year 2000, and 10 cm does not provide sufficient focus-to-object and focus-to-film/sensor distance for the proper employment of film holders (paralleling technique). The requirement for a large focus-to-object distance and large focus-to-film distance was discussed in Chapter 4 (imaging geometry Figure 4.7).

The step-up transformer has been discussed in previous chapters, and its function is to convert the 230 V mains supply to the kilovoltage that is required to generate X-rays (Chapter 2, Figure 2.3).

The step-down transformer converts the mains from 230 to 12 V for heating the filament so that the electron cloud that provides the electrons for the tube current can be released from its surface.

The tube housing is sealed so that the oil cannot leak and the air cannot enter; if either of these were to occur, there would be severe adverse effects on the electrical insulation.

The flexibility of the X-ray tube head is aided by the style of its mounting. They may be free standing on wheels so that they can be moved to other rooms, ceiling mounted or wall mounted. Whichever of these is used, the tube head is mounted on two or three lever arms that allow maximum reach and movement in both vertical and horizontal planes. The tube head is then mounted on two joints that also allow adjustment in vertical and horizontal directions.

Technical features

In Chapter 2 we saw that there are a range of voltage waveforms that could be employed in X-ray equipment.

Half-wave rectification in which half of the mains cycle is completely unused was often self-rectified (this means the X-ray tube provides the block to the reverse half cycle). This system is not particularly efficient or safe.

Full-wave rectification, in which a system of rectifiers inverts the negative half cycle, means the cathode and anode are always connected to the required electrical pole (negative or positive). In this system the negative half cycle is utilised, but there are long periods when the cathode and anode are connected to relatively low voltages and no useful X-rays will be produced.

Direct current, (constant or virtually constant potential) in these units the anode and cathode are always connected to the required pole; cathode –ve and anode +ve, and the potential is such that useful X-rays are produced throughout the cycle.

The tube current (electrons crossing the tube) in an intra-oral dental X-ray machine will be of the range 8–12 mA, that is 0.008–0.012 A.

The frequency of the mains supply is 50 cycles per second.

The kilovoltage will be either, 60, 65 or 70; there should be no 50 kV machines still in use as it was strongly advised that they be removed from clinical use by 2001.

The focal spot (focus) will be somewhere in the range $0.4–0.7 \, mm^2$ (this is of course the size of the apparent rather than actual focus (Chapter 4, Figure 4.1)).

The aluminium filter must meet minimum requirements, for X-ray equipment operating below 70 kV filtration must be at least 1.5 mm of aluminium and above 70 kV, 2.5 mm of aluminium. Total filtration in any X-ray system is calculated by adding inherent filtration to the added filtration. Inherent filtration is the filter effect on the beam provided by the fact that it has to pass through the glass envelope, mineral oil and the exit port. The added filtration is the aluminium placed either just inside or outside the exit port.

ORTHOPANTOMOGRAPHY

It is sometimes useful to be able to visualise all of the dentition at the same time; to do this with periapical images requires 10 or 12 exposures, and to do it with occlusal films would take five exposures. Either of these techniques is very invasive for the patient and time consuming for the staff.

In addition to the patient discomfort and staff time, there is the problem that there has to be very careful positioning of the films during the exposure followed by correct mounting to ensure that all of the teeth and surrounding structures will be shown clearly.

The alternative technique of pantomography is as the name suggests based on the theories of tomography.

To understand why we need tomography, we first have to look at one of the major limiting factors of general radiography. When producing a radiograph, we are trying to form an accurate image of a three-dimensional object in only two dimensions; there will always be a problem with structures that lie in front and behind the object that we are looking at. Imaging the mandible the overlying structure would be either the spine or the opposite side of the mandible (Figure 7.3). The arrows represent the X-ray beam.

> • If we take an image of the mandible from the back, the spine will overlie the image of the mandible and anterior teeth. If we take images of the mandible from either side, the opposite side of the mandible will lie over the detail that we wish to see.

Tomography is a technique that allows us to effectively blur out the detail of the structures that we do not want to see. The effect is achieved by the simultaneous movement of both the film and the X-ray tube.

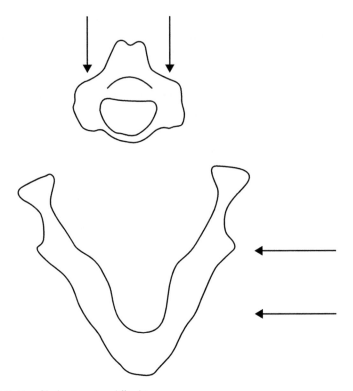

Figure 7.3 Mandibular imaging difficulties

If we imagine three structures within the patient at different levels, we can show the potential effect of this simultaneous movement of X-ray tube and film (Figure 7.4).

The three structures – triangle, star and X – are at different levels in the patient, and the movement of the X-ray tube and film is organised so that the centre of their turning circle (fulcrum) is at the level of the star.

With the X-ray tube at position A, all of the structures show superimposed in the middle of the film; from position B the star is still in the middle, but the X is on the far right of the film and the triangle on the left. When the structures are imaged from position C, the X is on the far left of the film and the triangle on the right.

The only structure that remains in the same place on the film is the star. The star will therefore be the only one of the three structures that will appear sharp on the image, and any other structure on the same level within the patient will also appear sharp.

The principle of tomography is quite simple, but when we start to think of the mandible, it becomes more complex because of its shape (Figure 7.5).

Looking at the general shape of the mandible (the maxilla will be similar), it is clear that there is not a single point that could be the centre of an arc (fulcrum) to cover all of the parts that we need to image. If the mandible and maxilla were a perfect semicircle, it would be possible.

The fact that the mandible effectively consists of two almost straight sides and a heavily curved centre means that three separate fulcrum points are needed during the exposure cycle. There is a separate fulcrum for each side of the mandible and one for the centre.

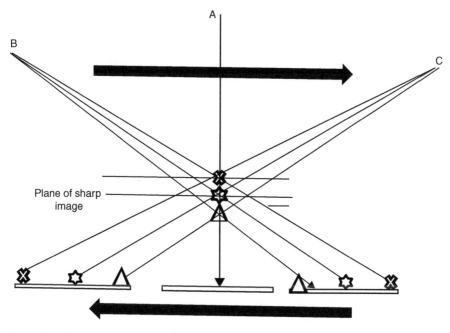

Figure 7.4 Tomographic imaging effect

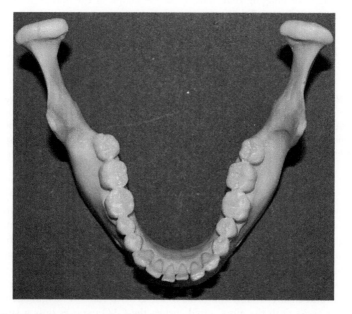

Figure 7.5 Mandibular tomography difficulties

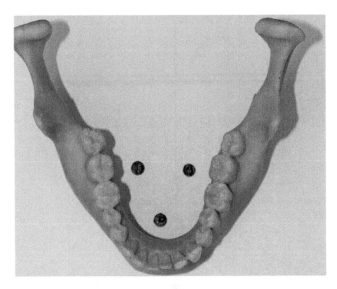

Figure 7.6 Pan-oral tomographic pivot points

The rotation centres (fulcrums) may be fixed points or continually moving to readjust to each part of the mandible; each manufacturer will have their own method of producing a sharp plane of imaging that matches to the shape of the mandible. Typical pivot points are shown in Figure **7.6**.

Fulcrum points for mandibular tomography

- The picture here (Figure 7.6) shows the three typical pivot points required to give a sharp image of the whole of the mandible. Because not all patients have the same shape of mandible or bite, the front (centre pivot point) is often adjustable (this is the focal trough). In some machines the pivot point is moved, and in others the patient is moved. Some even have a fixed focus to take in all mandibular outlines.

In Chapter 4 we discussed the importance of maintaining a film position parallel to the object that we are imaging and ensuring that the central ray of the X-ray beam is perpendicular (right angles) to the object and the film. The construction of the pantomography machines maintains these relationships between the beam, object and film for all parts of the mandible.

The construction of the OPG therefore provides a sharp plane of focus for all parts of the mandible and ensures that it conforms to the general rules of imaging geometry.

To further assist with the aims stated earlier, the OPG exposes only a small portion of the film/sensor at any particular instant. It does this by passing the beam through two small apertures, one close to the X-ray tube and one immediately in front of the image receptor (Figure 7.7).

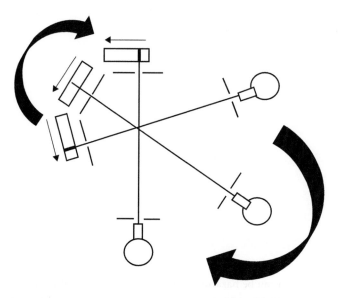

Figure 7.7 X-ray tube and film movement during pan-oral tomography

Tomographic imaging movement for OPTs

- As the film/sensor and X-ray tube rotate, the film slides along behind the exposure slot. In this way each part of the film is exposed only when the beam is at right angles to that area.

Here we see the effect of the two collimators; as the film/sensor rotates around the patient, it also moves across the holder that it is mounted in. The rotation matching that of the X-ray tube ensures that the X-ray beam is always at right angles to the film. The two collimators and the film sliding across the holder ensure that only that small part of the film that is at right angles to the beam is exposed in any instant. This arrangement follows the convention of placing the part being imaged parallel to the film and the centre of the beam being perpendicular to both the object and the image recorder (Figure 7.7).

An accurate image will be formed in this way.

Chapter 8

Radiation doses and dose measurement

UK POPULATION RADIATION DOSE

UK POPULATION RADIATION DOSE

Exposure to radiation can be hazardous to health, and as exposure increases, the potential for harm also increases. This means that it is important for us to know the level of dose that we are exposing people to when diagnostic radiographs are taken.

When investigating radiation doses to the UK population as a whole, total dose is separated into two main categories: natural background dose and man-made (or artificial) dose.

Background dose is derived from:

Cosmic rays from space
Gamma rays
Radon gas
Food and drink

Man-made dose is derived from a number of sources, some of which are obvious while others may be a little surprising; they are:

Medical and dental X-rays
Occupational
Fallout
Consumer products

Non-ionising radiation sources include:

Mobile phone
Microwave ovens
Microwave ovens and other appliances

Basic Guide to Dental Radiography, First Edition. Tim Reynolds.
© 2016 John Wiley & Sons, Ltd. Published 2016 by John Wiley & Sons, Ltd.

Medical and dental exposures

When all of the sources are taken into account, the total overall contribution to the UK population dose from background is approximately 83% and from man-made 17%. The majority of radiation dose to the UK population is therefore contributed by the sources that we are exposed to everyday and can't avoid with radon gas being the greatest single contributor.

Radon gas accounts for almost 50% of the total UK population annual dose.

What is important within the context of this text is the contribution to total dose that is made by medical and dental exposures.

When considering only artificial (man-made) sources, it accounts for approximately 90% of the total.

> • Information regarding UK population ionising radiations doses derived from HPA-RPD-001 May 2005. SJ Watson, AL Jones, WB Oatway and JS Hughes. Health Protection Agency Radiation Protection Division, Public Health England, The Stationery Office Limited.

The 90% of artificial exposure that is produced by medical and dental exposures is a very large proportion with medical and dental practitioners and operators having absolute control over the decision to deliver a radiation dose and the size of dose delivered.

When we make a further division of the dose sources, separating medical and dental, we find that general medical accounts for around 97% of the dose dental exposures for only 3% (these figures were taken from a time when full records were kept and do not take into account the growth in the use of cone beam computed tomography scanners in dental work).

The reasons for this large disparity become obvious when doses for individual examinations are investigated.

Everyone is used to the idea that a bitewing or periapical radiograph delivers the equivalent of around 8 h of background radiation dose and an OPG around 26 h.

These are much lower than some of the doses seen in general medical doses, for example, lower back (lumbar spine) delivers around 8 months' background equivalent and a computed tomography (CT) scan of the skull up to 1 year of background. Other CT scans deliver the equivalent of a few years of background radiation dose.

Doses in general medical X-ray examinations can therefore be many hundreds even thousands of times greater than those delivered during intra-oral or extra-oral examinations in dental practices.

This does not mean that the doses delivered in dental practices are insignificant because as we shall see later in this text, even the smallest of doses can have serious, even fatal, consequences.

DOSE MEASUREMENT

There are two characteristics of X-rays that allow us to measure the dose that has been delivered:

1. Ionisation
2. Excitation

RADIATION DOSES

Remember that ionisation is the removal of an electron from an atom and excitation is the temporary raising of an electron from its natural energy level to a higher one.

With ionisation we can assess dose by measuring the number of ionisations through the collection of negative charge or by observing the effect of ionisation on the atoms or molecules of the material that has been struck by the X-rays.

With excitation the dose is assessed by measuring the additional energy that has been deposited in the material.

TYPES OF DOSE METERS

The principal types of dose-measuring device are:

Free air ionisation chamber
Thimble ionisation chamber
Chemical conversion dose meter
Photographic density
Scintillation detectors
Semiconductor detectors
Calorimetry
Thermoluminescent dosimetry (TLD)

Some of these such as free air ionisation chamber, chemical conversion and calorimetry are laboratory methods only; they are used as primary standard dose meters for experimental work and for calibrating the dose meters used in practical situations. This is either because they are too large or simply require too closely controlled an environment for practical everyday use.

Others such as thimble ionisation chamber, photographic density and TLD are practical dose meters that may be used in your practice.

A thimble ionisation chamber may have been used to assess the dose delivered to your patients (that's if the measurement was performed by an engineer in the department).

Photographic density or TLD (usually TLD today) will be the method used to measure doses if the practice is one of those that monitor staff doses. The monitoring of staff doses is not a legal requirement except for those identified as classified persons.

A classified person is someone who is likely to receive 3/10s of their annual dose limit; this does not currently apply to anyone working in a dental practice.

THIMBLE IONISATION DOSE METER PICTURE

The device shown is an example of what would be called a thimble ionisation chamber (Figure 8.1). Electrons carrying negative charge are released in the chamber through ionisation. As the dose increases, the amount of charge released increases. The dose is shown by the deflection of the quartz fibre across a scale. Depending on the type the indicator will deflect from or collapse towards the central electrode.

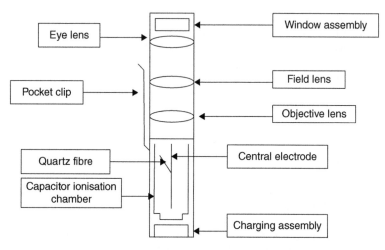

Figure 8.1 An example of a thimble ionisation dose meter (immediate readout)

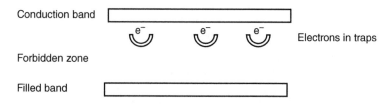

Figure 8.2 Dose recording on a TLD

Thermoluminescent dose meter: Thimble chamber

The most popular dose-measuring device for personnel monitoring is the TLD. It is worth taking a brief look at how the TLD works, particularly as it will seem familiar to you.

The molecules in a TLD material (lithium fluoride is a popular one) have a small number of electron traps in the forbidden zone between the outer electron energy levels. The material can be doped (have additional elements added) to increase the number of electron traps.

Following exposure to radiation, electrons undergoing excitation fall into the traps and maintain a record of the dose received as increased atom energy. As dose increases, the number of electrons in traps also increases, and energy stored in the atoms is raised in direct proportion to the dose received.

Thermoluminescent dose meter

Within a TLD material, after the dose has been delivered, there will be a number of electrons in traps; the number is directly proportional to the dose received, and the material is in a raised energy state (Figure 8.2).

The material will remain in this raised energy state for a considerable time; in fact the monitor is worn for up to 3 months, and with every additional dose received, more electrons are raised into traps so that the total dose over the whole period is recorded.

RADIATION DOSES

The electron traps are not, as shown in the diagram, actual cups but rather energy anomalies that hold the raised energy electrons.

It is now necessary to recover a reading of the dose that has been received by the person. To do this, the TLD is heated. The heating gives the electrons just enough energy to escape from the traps and fall back to their original energy level.

READING A TLD RECORD

After heating, the electrons shaken out of the traps have to give up the additional energy they have stored as they fall back to their original energy level. This additional energy is given up as visible light (Figure 8.3).

The amount of light given up is directly proportional to the number of electrons in traps which is in turn directly proportional to the dose received. Therefore the amount of light (intensity) given off is the indicator of how large a dose the person has received.

After the dose has been recorded, the TLD is further heated to totally remove any residual dose reading, and the TLD is ready to use again.

Before commencing on this brief explanation, I said it would be familiar, and if you glance back at Chapter 7, you will see that the process here is very similar to the operation of the phosphor plate image recording system.

The advantages of TLD dose monitoring over other methods are:

They are relatively inexpensive.

They are reusable, once the dose record has been erased.

They have a wide dynamic range (they can measure very small or quite large doses).

They are reasonably robust and resistant to physical damage.

The TLD material can be coated onto devices of a wide range of sizes (they can be used even in body cavities).

They are tissue equivalent (this means radiation is absorbed in exactly the proportion as it is in the human body).

They are able to measure both surface and deep tissue doses.

A major disadvantage of the TLD is that once it has been read, there is no permanent record of the dose received.

It is written down, but if there was a question about what had been written, you can't go back and check the TLD again because it will have been cleared for reuse.

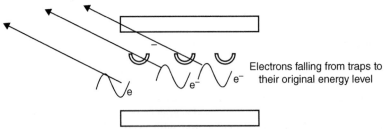

Light emitted as electrons fall to their original energy level

Electrons falling from traps to their original energy level

Figure 8.3 Thermoluminescent material, dose reading

Care must also be taken to keep them away from radiation sources and extremes of temperature as dose reading could be affected.

DOSE QUANTITIES

There are a number of different dose measurements that you might hear of, but we will discuss four here:

Radiation exposure
Absorbed dose
Dose equivalent
Effective dose

Radiation exposure

Rather than the dose delivered to the individual, exposure tells us how much radiation there is, that is, how many quanta passed through a particular area.

Exposure is measured in coulombs per kilogram (C/kg). You might be able to guess from this that exposure is assessed by measuring the number of ionisations that have taken place in a particular mass of material. It is measured by collecting the charge that has been displaced, by ionisation, from the atoms or molecules in that mass.

If the number of quanta passing through a mass of material is doubled, then the charge released will also be doubled.

Exposure is not a particularly useful measure as it tells us nothing of the interaction between the radiation and the material (tissue) that it is passing through. It tends to be a measure that is used to make comparisons between sources of radiation and to calibrate other dose meters.

Absorbed dose

This is a much more useful measurement than exposure because it actually tells us how much energy is absorbed by the person.

The amount of energy absorbed is important because the greater the energy deposited, the higher the risk of hazardous changes. Think of this in terms of the difference between giving someone a slight tap with your hand or a hard slap. The hand is the same, but the slap is much more damaging to the tissue because it deposits more energy.

Absorbed dose is assessed in terms of joules per kilogram (J/kg, joule is a general measure of energy). When measuring radiation absorbed dose instead of recording the dose as J/kg it is given the special name, 'the gray' (Gy); 1 gray is 1 J/kg.

Absorbed dose is the measurement most often used to assess patient doses in dental practices. There will be an assessment of patient dose in all dental practices as it is a legal requirement that those delivering medical and dental radiation doses to patients must be aware of the level of dose likely to be delivered.

The readings of patient dose for a dental practice for periapical or bitewing radiographs will be in the region of 0.7–2.0 milligray per square centimetre (mGy/cm^2).

It's worth making a special note here that for the majority of practices the dose will be recorded in this form and the patient dose is not, for example, 1 mGy but $1 mGy/cm^2$ of tissue exposed.

RADIATION DOSES

To find the true absorbed dose, you would need to take into account the area exposed. 1 mGy recorded but delivered to an area 5 cm × 5 cm produces a dose of 25 mGy.

Dose equivalent

This measurement of dose makes further efforts to make a more accurate assessment of the potential for harm to the person; it does this by adding in a radiation weighting factor. This additional factor is an expression of how dangerous the radiation is that the patient has been exposed to.

Examples of radiation weighting factors are:

Radiation type	Weighting factor
X-rays	1
Gamma rays	1
Electron beams	1
Proton and neutron beams	5–10 depending on energy
Alpha particles	20

Once this conversion has been made, the name of the unit is changed to sievert (Sv), so a dose from X-rays of 1 mGy/cm^2 is multiplied by a weighting factor of 1 to become 1 mSv.

Some engineering companies have dose meters that give a reading for dose that is expressed in terms of dose equivalent, so the numbers will look similar to those given earlier, but it will say sievert instead of gray.

Some of the meters also give more accurate readings if the recording is in terms of microgray or sievert (μ).

This can make the numbers look quite scary; remember that 700 μGy/cm^2 is 0.7 mGy/cm^2.

Effective dose

This is the most meaningful dose measurement in radiation safety terms because it is the only measurement that gives us a realistic assessment of the likely harm to the patient.

This accurate assessment is achieved by factoring in not only the radiation used but also the tissues exposed.

Full assessment of effective dose is given by multiplying the absorbed dose by the radiation weighting factor and then by weighting factors for tissues. The tissue weighting factors are divided into two groups, the core tissues and the remainder of the body.

Tissue weighting factors used in calculation of effective dose

Gonads
Stomach
Large bowel
Bone marrow
Lungs
Oesophagus
Liver
Thyroid
Bladder

Breast tissue
Skin
Bone surface
Salivary glands
Brain
Remainder of body

From: ICRP 2007. The 2007 Recommendations of the International Commission on Radiological Protection. ICRP Publication 103. Ann ICRP 37 (2–4).

The factor that links the majority of these tissues is a medium to high turnover and regeneration rate. Most cell damage is caused in the middle of the cell cycle when it is preparing for reproduction or at the point of reproduction (mitosis), so the more often the cells of a particular organ go through regeneration, the greater the chance of harm occurring.

If the absorbed dose used to calculate effective dose is in the form mGy/cm^2, then to complete the assessment, the area of tissue exposed must also be factored in.

The full calculation of effective dose would therefore be:

Absorbed dose × area exposed × radiation weighting factor × tissue weighting factors

This can be expressed as $Gy \times$ area exposed $\times W_R \times \Sigma\ W_T$

where
Gy = absorbed dose
W_R = weighting factor for radiation
W_T = weighting factor for tissues
Σ = the sum of

Effective dose gives us an accurate assessment of the potential for harm to the exposed person for all X-ray examinations.

The risk–benefit analysis that should always be performed before an X-ray examination is easier because we can calculate effective dose.

RADIATION DOSES

Chapter 9

Biological effects of X-rays

Following Roentgens discovery of X-rays in November 1895 and the production of the first radiograph, there was a rapid development of this new diagnostic science. Initially little attention was paid to safety aspects as the X-rays were regarded as simply another kind of light.

There were reports of burns in both patients and operators and in some cases a degree of nausea; the most severe cases were seen among those working with the X-rays as the X-ray tubes were open to the air and the staff were exposed constantly.

However even severe burns were seen to heal and in reasonable time, it was believed that there were no long-term harmful effects. This belief was so widely held that in America a clinician was asked if he may be able to demonstrate with X-rays a bullet in the skull of a child. Not being sure he placed a coin on one of his associates' heads and exposed him to radiation for 1 h. No image of the coin was seen, and 21 days later the associate lost his hair. Far from identifying this as a sign of real hazard, the news was given that for men X-rays could make shaving a thing of the past.

This lax state ended in 1904 with a number of, seemingly X-ray-related deaths. Over the following years more was written about the safety aspects of diagnostic X-rays, and in 1928 the first committee with a remit to investigate radiation safety was formed.

In 1939 a memorial to 'the X-ray martyrs' was erected at Hamburg University; it listed 169 names. By 1959 the list numbered 352. These martyrs were X-ray workers who had died as a result of the effects of radiation.

Although radiographs do provide an extremely useful diagnostic aid, it must be remembered that there is also hazard in their use and this must always be kept in mind when radiographs are requested and produced.

In Chapter 3, page 27, we discussed atomic structure in relation to X-ray interactions; you will remember that we said all atoms consist almost entirely of free space. We also said that in relation to the limited solid particle mass and the amount of free space, an X-ray quantum is tiny so that the greatest likelihood is that quanta will miss the solid material and pass through the space.

This is as true in human tissue as it is in any other medium. It follows then that during any X-ray examination large numbers of quanta may pass through the patient without contacting any of the particles making up the atoms within the tissues.

Basic Guide to Dental Radiography, First Edition. Tim Reynolds.
© 2016 John Wiley & Sons, Ltd. Published 2016 by John Wiley & Sons, Ltd.

Despite the statements made previously, there will be many contacts between X-ray quanta and particles in the patient simply because of the very high numbers of quanta involved. Each of the quanta will be capable of producing many ionisations because they carry much more energy than that required to liberate an electron from human tissue.

Even if only a very small percentage of the quanta strike solid particles in the body, there will be very large numbers of ionised atoms. The chemical properties of the atoms will be changed by the removal of an electron through ionisation and the subsequent rearranging of electron positions within the shells of the atom.

The whole process is one of random chance; in addition to atoms being mostly free space, the electrons are moving in orbits around the nucleus, and the X-ray quanta are moving through the atom at the speed of light. For an interaction to take place, the electron and the quantum must arrive at exactly the same point at exactly the same time. (It's like knowing your best friend will be in London shopping on a particular day but you don't know where, but you go to London hoping to bump into them having made no arrangements.)

Given this idea of random chance, what are the quanta most likely to interact with? The answer is, of course, whatever is present in the greatest quantities; most of you will know that in most living things the most abundant material is water. In childhood our body is around 70% water, and as an adult it falls to around 60% although some tissues may be as high as 90% water. For an adult of around 72 kg weight, this means 45 litres of water (this is a lot of water).

This abundance of water means that it is the molecule most likely to interact with the X-ray quanta passing through. The chemistry of radiation effects on water is therefore very important to this subject of radiobiology.

We must just take a time out here to remind ourselves that this text is a basic guide. Radiobiology is a large and complex subject, and detailed study does not fall within the scope of our aim. We will be looking at the basis of these X-ray interactions, but the explanations will be well short of fully detailed chemical and biological analysis of the process.

INDIRECT EFFECTS OF RADIATION DOSES

There cannot be many people that don't know that the chemical symbol for water is H_2O, two hydrogen atoms and one oxygen atom. In this water molecule the negative charges (electrons) and positive charges (protons) are in balance, so the molecule has no overall negative or positive charge.

Following ionisation by an X-ray quantum, the water molecule having lost an electron is no longer balanced in terms of its electric charges; the removal of a unit of negative charge leaves the molecule with a positive charge.

Putting in some straightforward numbers, we are saying that if there were originally 10 electrons and 10 protons in a molecule, it would be electrically neutral. If you take away an electron, you have 9 negative and 10 positive charges, so overall the molecule will be slightly positive.

There will also be a high-speed electron moving through the medium; it has been removed from its position in one of the shells in the molecule and given a large amount of kinetic energy (energy of movement).

We can show this in a simple chemical flow chart.

Fast moving electron with negative charge

$$H_2O + X\text{-ray quantum} \longrightarrow H_2O^+ + e^-$$

Water molecule with positive charge

The electron will move through the material giving up the kinetic energy in interactions with other molecules as it travels through the medium.

As it slows, it is likely to be captured by another water molecule; this molecule also then has an electrical imbalance, but it is in the opposite direction, and it has an additional electron so it has an overall negative charge:

$$H_2O + e^- \rightarrow H_2O^-$$

A normal electrically neutral water plus an electron produces a negatively charged water molecule.

As a result of this process, we now have two 'abnormal' water molecules – one with a negative charge and one with a positive charge.

Both of these molecules are unstable (remember Chapter 1, pages 5 on the role of electrons in joining atoms together).

The unstable molecules dissociate (fall apart). This results in the formation of an ion (charged particle) and a free radical:

$$H_2O^+ \rightarrow H^+ + \overset{\bullet}{O}H$$

$$H_2O^- \rightarrow \overset{\bullet}{H} + OH^-$$

The dot above the OH in the first example and the H in the second example denotes that these are free radicals. These free radicals may go through large numbers of subsequent reactions either with other water molecules, with the products of the first dissociation or with biological molecules.

These interactions can lead to radiobiological effects.

Damage that occurs in this way is generally termed indirect damage. The biological molecules have been damaged by chemical changes following the interactions between the radiation and water molecules, not radiation and the biological molecule.

The route to actual biological damage through the ionisation of water molecules is more complex than the one outlined but this brief explanation is sufficient for this text.

DIRECT BIOLOGICAL EFFECTS OF RADIATION DOSES

The radiation quantum hits the critical biological molecule and ionises it.

$$BM + \text{radiation} \longrightarrow BM^+ + e^- \longrightarrow \overset{\bullet}{B} + M^+$$

Biological molecule

BIOLOGICAL EFFECTS OF X-RAYS

After ionisation the biological molecule has a positive charge and there is a free electron.

Just as with the ionisation of the water molecule, the ionisation of the biological molecule destabilises it, and it dissociates to form the free radical.

The end result of the biological damage may be the same regardless of the damage being done directly or indirectly. Ionisations do not generally occur as single event but in clusters. These ionisations are the principal cause of radiation effects in living tissue.

The damage produced by ionisation may be seen in biological macromolecules such as DNA, RNA and enzymes, or it could be seen in cytoplasmic organelles such as mitochondria or lysosomes and cell membranes.

So we now know that biological tissues can be affected either directly by radiation (if the quanta hit a significant biological molecule) or indirectly when the quanta hit water molecules and the chemical changes that follow have adverse effects on the biological molecules. Direct and indirect effects will have the similar end results for the tissues/person involved.

The effects discussed so far in this chapter are at molecular and subcellular levels: molecular in the ionisation of water molecules and DNA and subcellular in the case of effects on mitochondria, lysosomes and cell membranes.

Next we must consider the potential effects on the cells themselves.

As with many of the subjects we have studied in this text, the effects on radiation on cells are a large and complex subject well beyond what is required for basic understanding. For the purposes of this study, we will content ourselves with the inclusion of only the headlines of cellular effects.

There are four potential outcomes for cells following exposures to radiation:

1. Complete repair: The human body has great capacity to repair itself following all types of damage. This capacity extends to radiation damage, and as a result not all of the damage caused by radiation exposure is irreversible. The cell may repair and continue to function and reproduce as normal.
2. Cell death: The immediate halting of all normal function and subsequent decomposition is how we would define death. This type of death does occur in cells and the term generally applied to this is interphase cell death (interphase because death occurs before the cell can reach its next reproductive event).
3. Prevention of cell reproduction: Here the cell affected continues to function normally, but when it completes the cycle to what would be its reproductive phase, the process is not triggered and there is no cell division (no mitosis). This type of effect may be referred to as mitotic death.
4. Mutation: This occurs when a cell has damage that does not repair or repairs incompletely before reproduction. At reproduction the information passed to the new daughter cells includes the original damage or the incorrect repair. The result is new 'daughter' cell that has defects. When the daughter cells reproduce, the defect is passed to subsequent cell generations; this may later develop into clinically significant changes.

We now consider the effects of radiation damage on tissues, organs and the whole being; we can look into these effects as two distinct different categories.

These categories are stochastic effects and deterministic effects.

STOCHASTIC EFFECTS OF RADIATION EXPOSURE

The most often used example for stochastic effects is the radiation-induced fatal or non-fatal tumour; the main characteristics of these effects are as follows:

1. They are random and unpredictable. This means we do not know who will be affected or the level of dose at which the effect will become apparent. Some individuals will show this type of effect at comparatively low doses, while others having received significant doses show no obvious effect. It is important to indicate at this point that we are not saying that if there is no obvious effect, there has been no radiation damage; it is just that there has been no clinically observable sign or symptom.
2. Although random and unpredictable, we know that the probability of developing a stochastic effect increases linearly as dose increases. This is generally true regardless of whether the dose is delivered as a single large dose or of many repeated smaller doses.
3. There is no threshold dose; this means that there is no dose below which these effects definitely cannot occur. The opposite is also true; There is no dose at which we can guarantee the effect will occur.
4. The severity of the effect is not dose or dose rate related (dose rate is how quickly the dose is delivered). This means that a small dose does not mean a mild effect and a large dose does not mean a severe effect. The factor that governs the severity is the site or tissue or organ where the effect becomes apparent.
5. There is no repair process; any dose delivered therefore always has the potential to cause actual harm at some point in later life.
6. The effects are accumulative; that is, generally every dose adds to the potential for harm that has been produced by every previous dose; it is therefore the total dose over any period (including whole lifetime) that governs the probability of developing a stochastic effect.

We can pull together the final two points given previously with the statement:
'There is no such thing as a safe waiting time between X-ray examinations'. Radiographs cannot be taken on the basis on the time elapsed since the last one was taken. It must always be a decision taken on clinical, not chronological, grounds.

DETERMINISTIC OR NON-STOCHASTIC EFFECTS

In this category we are considering effects such as radiation burns, cataracts and temporary sterility in men. In many ways the effects that fall into this category are the opposite in terms of the characteristics of those that are stochastic.

The characteristics of these effects are as follows:

1. There is a threshold dose above which there is an increasing probability that the effect will occur but below which it will not.
2. Severity is to some extent dependent on the dose and the dose rate, so the greater the dose, the worse the effect.
3. There is some recovery process between successive doses.
4. The effects are only partially accumulative; the increasing risk does not vary arithmetically as dose increases.

BIOLOGICAL EFFECTS OF X-RAYS

WHO WILL BE AFFECTED

When looking at where these radiation effects fall, there are two categories for persons affected: somatic effects and genetic effects.

Somatic effects are quite simply those that occur in an irradiated individual (the person who is hit by the radiation is the one who has the health problem). Somatic effects may be either stochastic or deterministic.

Genetic effects: Most people will realise immediately that we are considering effects that will occur in future generations. These effects occur as a result of damage to germ cells and will always be stochastic.

Radiation-induced biological detriment will change depending on the age of the person at the point of exposure. The younger a person is when they are exposed, the greater the hazard. The most critical age group is from ages 1 to 10 years; exposure during this period is approximately twice as hazardous as it would be for an adult.

DETRIMENT WITH AGE AT EXPOSURE

- The histogram shown in Figure 9.1 gives only a general idea of the relative risk. Children of 10 years and under have a risk of around double than that of someone in their 30s (Wall BF, Haylock R, Jansen JTM, Hiller M, Hart D and Shrimpton PC. HPA-CRCE-028. Relative Risk for Medical X-ray Examinations as a Function of Age and Sex of the Patient. Chilton: HPA; 2011).

There are a number of reasons for the differences demonstrated in this bar chart:

1. In the earlier age groups, there are more cells undergoing rapid regeneration.
2. There is a much greater probability that those exposed early in their life will live long enough for late-onset radiation effects to become apparent.

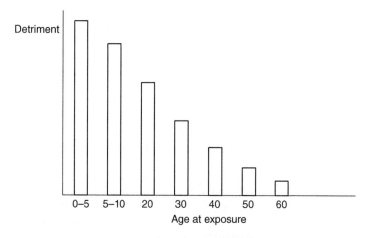

Figure 9.1 Radiation detriment, variations with age at exposure

BIOLOGICAL EFFECTS OF X-RAYS

3. There are tissues that are still differentiating (coming to their final form); any radiation damage during this time will be passed on to later generations of cells of the particular type.

Whole body sensitivity to radiation depends on many factors including:

Total dose
Type of radiation
Age at exposure
Type of cell
Current position in cell cycle
Total volume of tissue exposed
Body area exposed (trunk, extremity, etc.)
Period of exposure
Current state of health

When all risk factors are taken into account, it is possible to estimate the risk for any examination with a good degree of accuracy.

Not all texts will quote the same figures, but for dental radiography, the risk of fatal consequences from an intra-oral exposure may be around 1 in 3 million; for an OPG it may be in the region of 1 in every million examinations.

All of the information given throughout this chapter tells us that although the radiograph is an extremely useful diagnostic aid, it must be used only when absolutely necessary. When it is used, those performing the examination must do whatever is possible to reduce the dose delivered to the patient.

There must always be a risk–benefit analysis with the positive result, that is, the potential benefit to the patient must be greater than the risks.

It is also important to ensure that the doses for those working with radiation are as low as they can be and wherever possible there should be no dose at all as there is no such thing as a safe dose of radiation. Even the smallest dose will cause some ionisation and subsequent liberation of free radicals, leading to the abnormal chemical reactions that could cause clinically significant changes.

Following the previous statement, it is essential that we protect people from excessive or unnecessary radiation doses.

DOSE REDUCTION FOR PATIENTS

Ways in which the dose to patients can be reduced would include:

Only take radiographs that have clear clinical justification.
Carefully check the identification of the patient (to ensure a patient does not have the wrong examination).
Check the patients' symptoms (do the symptoms match the requested examination).
Ask about recent X-ray examinations at other practices (records must be transferred; you cannot take a new radiograph simply because an old record has not been transferred).
Ensure all relevant quality checks have been made on X-ray and accessory equipment (this will avoid repeats due to equipment faults).

BIOLOGICAL EFFECTS OF X-RAYS

Use film holders to minimise the number of repeat examinations due to errors.

Make use of high kV techniques wherever possible. (This produces scatter that travels in a more forward direction rather than up and down through other tissues.)

Use the fastest film available. EF is recommended. (This reduces the dose required to produce sufficient density to make the diagnosis.)

Wherever possible make use of rectangular collimators. (Don't do this if it will increase the chance of having to repeat the examination due to missing information, that is, patients who are likely to move)

DOSE REDUCTION FOR STAFF

Methods would include:

Minimise the number of staff members who will be in the vicinity of the X-ray equipment during examinations.

Make sure that all staff are made aware of the potential hazards.

Ensure that controlled areas are correctly defined and that there is a safe place for operators to stand during the procedure.

Make sure that barriers between radiation areas and adjacent work or rest areas provide sufficient protection.

Ensure that all safety checks on X-ray equipment are completed on schedule.

Perform radiation dose monitoring for staff (this cannot of course prevent the first accidental exposure, but subsequent investigation should reveal the source and prevent any further exposures). Remember that this is not specifically required.

Chapter 10

Legislation: Ionising Radiations Regulations 1999 (IRR 1999)

IRR 1999 is one of the two sets of regulations that were passed into law in the United Kingdom in the year 2000, and the second was the 'Ionising Radiations (Medical Exposures) Regulations 2000'. IRR 1999 was introduced into law on 1 January 2000, and IR(ME)R on 1 May 2000. These regulations were introduced in response to a document published in January of 1990; that document was ICRP 60(90), that is, International Commission for Radiation Protection document 60 of 1990.

This document readdressed the risks posed by exposures to ionising radiations; in broad terms the document indicated that all medical/dental exposure had risk factors three times greater than had previously been thought.

In response to ICRP 60(90) the European Commission (EC) published new Basic Safety Standards and EURATOM directives indicating the required elements for new regulations to be introduced across all member states of the European Union.

The two sets of regulations introduced in 2000 are enforced under the Health and Safety at Work Act 1974. The Health and Safety at Work Act makes everyone in any workplace responsible for their own safety and the safety of their colleagues and any other person who comes into the workplace for any purpose.

This means that everyone who works in any dental practice is responsible in some measure for radiation safety in that workplace; the level of responsibility will depend on the tasks that they perform within the practice.

IONISING RADIATIONS REGULATIONS 1999 (STATUTORY INSTRUMENT 3232)

An important point to note regarding these regulations is that they do not protect patients; in fact the patient is not mentioned in the documentation although some of the regulatory requirements will be of benefit to the patient.

The regulations contained within IRR 1999 cover four key areas:

1. Does this radiation workplace provide a safe working environment?
2. Is everything possible being done to protect those who work here?
3. Are there adequate protection measures in place for members of the public?
4. Is this workplace able to demonstrate adequate management of radiation protection?

Basic Guide to Dental Radiography, First Edition. Tim Reynolds.
© 2016 John Wiley & Sons, Ltd. Published 2016 by John Wiley & Sons, Ltd.

The regulations also cover the need to introduce a comprehensive quality assurance for all of the primary and accessory equipment used in the production of a radiograph.

The regulations that have a direct bearing on the processes in a dental practice are as follows.

Notification of specified work

All new dental practices must inform the Health and Safety Executive of the intention to open a practice and to use ionising radiation. This notification must be entered at least 28 days before the practice opens, and it must detail the work to be undertaken with radiation.

An acknowledgement of this notification must be received from the executive.

Notification and acknowledgement must be in place before a practice can legally use radiation. If no acknowledgement of the notification is received, the practice should make further representations to the executive.

During any inspection the inspectors generally wish to see the acknowledgement, not the original notification.

Risk assessment

Every room in which there is an X-ray unit must have its own bespoke risk assessment document. Risk assessment documents must be written specifically for each room because the doors, windows and X-ray machines will all be in different positions and walls may be of different construction.

Example:

In surgery, as shown here, the X-ray beam will be directed towards the window when doing left side periapical or bitewing radiographs and towards the door when doing right side. For anterior radiographs the beam will be directed towards the wall between surgeries 1 and 2 (Figure 10.1).

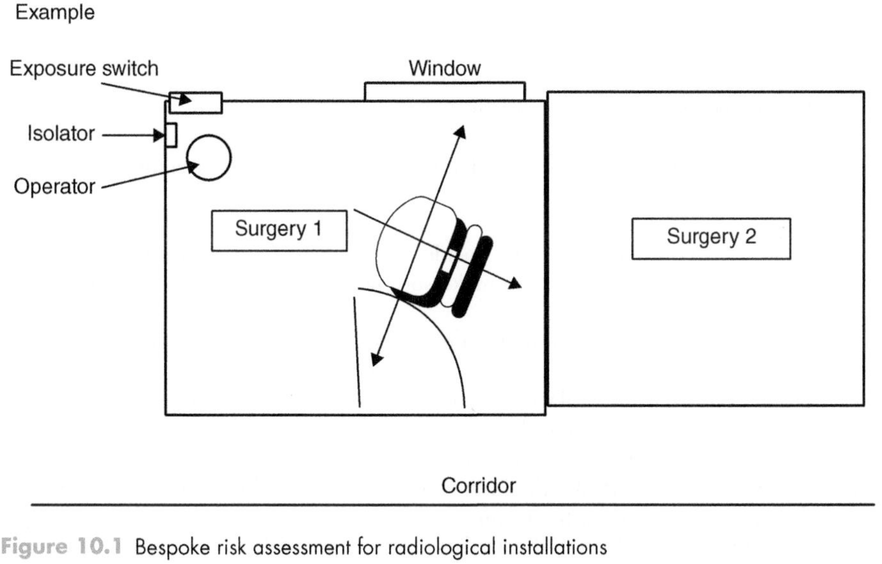

Figure 10.1 Bespoke risk assessment for radiological installations

Factors that need to be considered are as follows:

When the beam points towards the window, does it present any risk to anyone, and if so, what can and will be done to minimise or eliminate that risk?

When investigating risk, the existence of and level of risk will depend on what is on the other side of the window and the level of dose outside the window.

If the window is on the first floor and overlooks the back of the practice with no other buildings in close proximity, there is no risk.

If the window is on the ground floor and there is public access, it must be assumed that people will be at risk, and safety measures to minimise that risk must be put in place. Unless there is no dose outside the window.

When the beam points towards the door, what can be done to actively prevent someone walking through the door at the point of making the exposure? The operator cannot exclude anyone because they are positioned at the far side of the room and have no direct control over entry through the door.

When the beam points towards the wall of surgery 2, there will be some risk to those working or being treated there unless the wall provides a safe barrier to radiation penetration.

This means knowing two things:

1. What is the construction of the wall (double brick, single brick, block, stud partition)?
2. Is there any added radiation protection material if required (barium plaster, lead sheet, etc.)?

When the beam points towards the wall of the corridor outside the surgery:

1. Is the wall a safe barrier?
2. Is any necessary added radiation safety material in place?

When all of these questions have been answered, the level of risk will have been adequately assessed:

1. Is there a risk?
2. What is the size of the risk (level of potential exposure)?
3. How many people are likely to be affected?

Next we have to answer the question, 'what can be done to reduce or eliminate the risk?' In the case of the corridor:

1. Lead lining or barium plaster could be added to make the barrier adequate.
2. Measures could be put in place to make sure no one was in the corridor during the exposure.
3. The patient could be turned to make sure the beam does not point towards that wall.

Where measures are put in place to restrict access (other than by warning lights) or to modify radiation beam directions, the measures must be described in writing.

These written safety directions may be placed in the local rules for this room or in a specific scheme of work. Ideally the instructions for safe working specific to any room should be clearly displayed in that room.

A copy should also be filed in the 'Radiation Protection File'.

LEGISLATION

Restriction of exposure

This regulation indicates that employers must do all that is reasonably practicable to reduce doses to their staff. This will include ensuring that all engineering controls, warning devices and protective equipment are in good order and properly used at all times. It also requires that there are adequate schemes of work to ensure safe working practices.

It also means being sure that any wall between radiation-producing equipment and an adjacent working or rest area is an adequate barrier, that is, if the primary field of radiation is ever directed towards that barrier.

Personal protective equipment

This equipment (lead rubber aprons would be included) must conform to EC standards, and instruction must be given covering appropriate and proper use.

The correct type of housing must be provided for when it is not in use, and there must be periodic testing into its continued effectiveness.

Some questions arising from this might be the following:

Does the practice have lead rubber aprons?
   Are they stored correctly? They should hang perfectly straight over a large hanger; the only position in which they should bend is across the top of the shoulders.
   Folding or bending creates cracks and low-density spots making the apron less effective for its purpose.

What was the date of its last safety audit test?
   Testing of aprons is performed on closed-circuit X-ray TV systems such as those used for barium studies in hospitals; cracks and low-density areas that would let radiation through would be highlighted. If these areas are excessive, the apron may be condemned.
   There should be a schedule indicating the date of the last and next test. If this testing is not carried out, the apron cannot be used to protect persons because you cannot guarantee its effectiveness. No specific time period is suggested for retesting.

What is its appropriate use?
   Should lead rubber aprons be given to patients? The short answer to this is, 'No, why would they be appropriate?'
   In Chapter 9 we saw that the most important of our dose-measuring quantities is 'effective dose'.
   We also saw that an important part of the calculation is the contribution to dose provided by internal scattering of quanta of radiation.
   The next question is, 'what can a lead apron do to prevent or reduce the amount of internal scatter?'
   The answer is of course 'nothing'.
   The effective dose to the patient is likely to remain the same regardless of the use of a lead rubber apron.
   Modern X-ray equipment provides levels of safety that mean little or no radiation will pass directly down from the tube housing to the patient; this is the only type of dose that an apron would protect against.

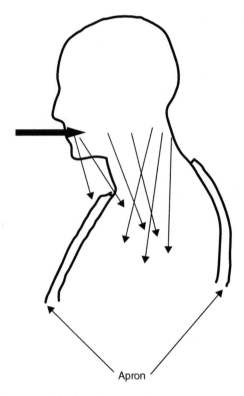

Apron

Figure 10.2 Internal scatter and lead rubber protection

The apron would therefore be providing protection from a radiation dose that is highly unlikely to occur with modern equipment (Figure 10.2).

- The heavy-filled arrow in figure 10. 2 represents the X-ray beam entering the mouth to produce an image of the upper central incisors. The smaller arrows show scattered rays passing down through the body to impact on critical organs within the body.
- This is where the majority of the radiation dose to the patient is derived.
- It is clear from the diagram that placing a lead rubber apron around the patient will have little or no effect on the total dose received. The bulky and uncomfortable apron may in fact cause the patient to move necessitating an additional exposure.

Dose limitation

This regulation sets the specific dose limits for those working with or around ionising radiations. From personal experience, reading many sets of local rules or radiation protection files, I have found that many dental practices adopt incorrect dose limits for their staff.

Radiographers working in hospitals have an annual dose limit of 20 mSv per year with an investigation level of one third of this (6 mSv).

Investigation level means that if a member of staff receives this dose, an investigation into the source must be undertaken to ensure that further doses are prevented in order that they do not reach the dose limit.

Given that patient doses in dental practices are very much smaller than those delivered in hospitals, the potential level for staff dose is also very much lower.

The annual dose limit suggested as appropriate for dental workers aged 18 and over working with X-ray is 1 mSv per year.

It is important to note (if you read the full regulations) that the staff described here are not 'classified persons'. Those who are designated as classified persons are workers who are likely to receive three tenths of their annual dose limit.

If a dental practice is designed and operated within the regulations and guidelines for ionising radiations, it is highly unlikely that any member of staff will receive three tenths of their dose limit and the designation of classified persons is not necessary.

If there are members of staff under 18 or who will never work with or near the radiation equipment (e.g. someone whose work involved reception desk duties only), there is a much lower suggested dose limit of 0.3 mSv per year.

These limits are whole-body effective dose limits.

Contingency plans

Contingency plans must be drawn up so that everyone knows what must be done in the case of a radiation accident.

Many people would think that radiation accidents do not occur in dental practices.

An accident however is any fault that occurs in an X-ray unit while it is in use. When using this definition for an accident, they are a reasonably regular occurrence; most will not result in any excessive dose to the patient. However, in some cases there may be significant increases in the dose delivered.

- An example would be. The exposure terminates prematurely producing a low density image, the examination must be repeated. The cause of the low density image must be investigated.

If the film was inserted the right way round, correct exposure settings used and the processor working then the fault lies with the X-ray machine.

In the event of accidents, in addition to the immediate actions noted in the local rules a full investigation involving all of those involved should be initiated.

The purpose of this investigation is to identify the reasons for the occurrence and prevent similar future events.

Should an investigation reveal an increase in patient dose of 20 times or more over that which is expected official notification is required (Health and Safety Executive for equipment failures and Care Quality Commission Medical Exposures Directorate for failures in procedures.

A note should be made in the patients' notes and the patient informed.

A second exposure was required, so there is an increase in the overall expected dose, a small initial dose is added to the correct second exposure.

- The machine may fail to terminate the exposure. This can result in quite significant dose increases, particularly if staff members are unaware of the correct actions or if the mains isolator is not correctly positioned, close to where the operator stands to initiate the exposure.

LEGISLATION

- An OPG machine may stall in the middle of its movement (it simply stops moving) with some OPG machines, particularly older types; if this happens, the exposure does not terminate, so the patient is receiving dose with no diagnostic information being gained.

Everyone concerned with the operation of the X-ray machines must know exactly what to do in any of these events.

Contingency plans for immediate action do not have to be very detailed. For major events the (RPA) will be fully involved in the investigation and will make an assessment of dose to the patient.

The immediate action contingency plans should be contained within the local rules, and they will contain three simple statements.

In case of accident:

- Immediately switch off the mains supply.
- Notify the RPA (only necessary if you suspect there has been excessive dose). You can discuss the circumstances of the accident, and the RPA can decide if there is any need for a visit to investigate and assess the patients' dose.
- A note should be put on the machine saying it is faulty and must not be used again until it is checked by an engineer. This is because if there is a small fault that occasionally causes the retaking of a radiography, there is ongoing overdosing of patients, and it must not be allowed.

Radiation protection advisors (RPA)

Prior to 1 January 2000 there was no need for dental practices to appoint a Radiation Protection Advisor (RPA) because under the old regulations (Ionising Radiations Regulations 1985), there was a special order (Exemption Order number 1, 1986).

The order exempted dental practices from the appointment of an RPA, and this was allowed because in general doses in dentistry are very low.

However ICRP 60(90) with the increased risk estimates changed this and IRR1999 requires that an RPA is appointed to all practices.

The RPA:

- Must be an external advisor (it cannot be anyone who works in the practice)
- Must be appointed in writing
- Must be appropriately qualified and of sufficient standing to carry out their duties
- Has to be regularly re-accredited (this can be checked on the Health and Safety Executive website)

In the case of a new practice, the appointment must be made before the practice opens so that advice can be given on setting up the practice properly. The employer must provide sufficient information to the RPA for them to perform their task properly.

The RPA should be consulted on all matters relating to IRR1999, for example:

- HSE notification
- Risk assessment
  - Contingency plans
  - Critical examination of equipment
- Local rules
- Dose limits
- Adequate barriers

- Quality assurance programmes
  - Specific delineated limits for controlled areas

Information and training

This regulation sets out requirements for basic safety training; you will remember that everyone in the practice is to some extent responsible for radiation safety. The level of responsibility will change as more specific and demanding tasks related to radiography are designated to a member of staff.

At the basic level people will be responsible for themselves, their colleagues and other persons in the same vicinity.

Those working in radiation workplaces must be aware of:

The nature of ionising radiations
The health risks presented by exposure
Radiation protection measures
Their responsibilities under the regulations (technical and administrative)
All restricted areas and times of restriction

Designation of controlled areas

A controlled area is effectively an exclusion zone around an X-ray unit to prevent unnecessary or excessive doses to any person in the general vicinity.

It is a legal requirement that an area around the equipment is designated as controlled and that it should be clearly demarcated (identified).

Many people use a loose definition of the controlled area as being anywhere close to the X-ray machine; although this is a reasonable statement for general purposes, it does not qualify as accurately defined and demarcated.

The controlled area will be anywhere that it is possible for a person to receive three tenths of their annual dose limit or where the instantaneous dose rate exceeds $7.6\,\mu Sv/h$ (7.6 microsievert per hour).

All is very well, but what does it mean in practical terms for a dental practice?

The actual size of the controlled area will depend on the maximum energy of the quanta in the X-ray beam. There are two categories for describing controlled areas in dental practices: X-ray machines operating below 70 kV and X-ray machines operating at or above 70 kV.

One very important point to remember is that the controlled area is not circular; you cannot stand anywhere near as close to an X-ray unit if you are in front of it as you can if you are behind it.

Below 70 kV the controlled area extends for 1 m round the X-ray tube and patient, and at or above 70 kV, the controlled area is 1.5 m round the X-ray tube or patient. In each of these cases, above and below 70 kV, the controlled area continues in the path of the primary beam (or in the direction of the primary beam) until it is attenuated by either a physical barrier or sufficient distance. These measurements are not used if the whole room is designated as a controlled area.

Controlled areas at below and above 70 kV

Figure 10.3a shows the stated measurements of controlled areas at 60 or 65 kV and at 70 kV; the major discussion point that comes up is the definition of the two statements (in the path of the primary beam and in the direction of the primary beam).

LEGISLATION

(a)

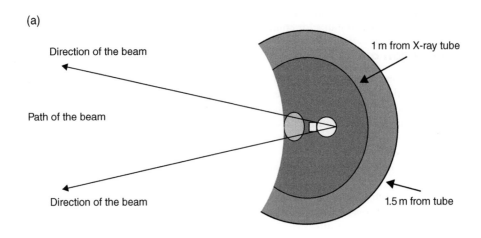

(b)

Distinction between in the path of or in the direction of is:

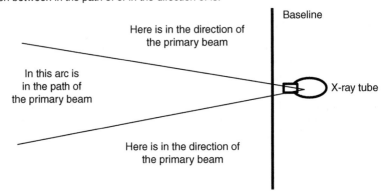

Figure 10.3 (a) Designated controlled areas. (b) Determination of controlled areas

The distinction between in the path of the primary beam and in the direction of the primary beam is the following:

In the path of means in the actual arc covered by the primary radiation beam (around 30–35°)
In the direction of means anywhere in front of the line labelled baseline (Figure 10.3b)

The general advice given is that the operator should stand 2 m from and behind the X-ray tube; that would mean 2 m behind the line labelled baseline and nowhere in front of it, unless there is a physical barrier that provides adequate radiation protection (Figure 10.4).

If there is no physical barrier, the statement that says 'or sufficient distance' is not relevant as it is not possible to stand far enough away to be considered perfectly safe in any dental surgery.

Whether your controlled area is defined by the statement 'continues in the path of the primary beam' or 'continues in the direction of the primary beam', the safe option is to follow the general advice and make sure that you are always behind the line labelled baseline in Figure 10.3b.

Advised safe standing area

This figure (10.4) shows the stated extent of the controlled area.

The line labelled 1 m from the patient and X-ray tube shows the stated controlled area for X-ray machines working at 60 or 65 kV.

The marked line is 1.5 m from the X-ray tube and patient and represents the stated controlled area for a dental X-ray machine operating at or above 70 kV. The semicircle marked 2 m is where the operator is advised to stand.

In both cases the figure shows an absolute exclusion zone (in the path of the primary beam) and an advised exclusion zone (in the direction of the primary beam). In the area of advised exclusion, there will be scattered quanta that are travelling in the general direction of the primary beam; these quanta will be high-energy quanta and still potentially capable of multiple ionisations.

The semicircle enclosed with the heavy black line represents the area 2 m from and behind the X-ray tube, the area in which operators are advised to stand during the exposure.

Other consideration for controlled areas

Restrictions of access to the controlled area

Only the patient is allowed in the controlled area during the exposure. The exception to this rule is for patients who are unable to comply with your instructions; the reasons for this may be age related or due to physical or mental disability.

LEGISLATION

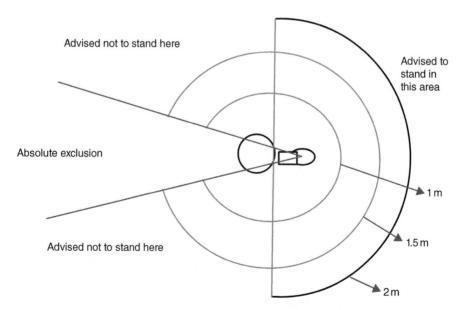

Figure 10.4 Designated controlled areas and advice on operator position

When we take radiographs, we want to obtain a good result at the first exposure; if the patients' condition makes this difficult, a carer is allowed into the controlled area to provide assistance.

Where this is necessary, the person acting as the carer should not be a member of staff.

This is because staff members are working in a radiation environment all the time and there is always some chance that they will receive an unnecessary dose of radiation; placing them in a position close to the patient would increase these chances unacceptably.

Note that we say staff *should not* rather than *must not* as there will be occasions when there is no alternative to a member of staff performing this function.

The carer should be a sensible adult person who accompanied the patient to the practice. Instruction should be given indicating exactly what is required of them, and the small but still present risk must be discussed with them.

Every effort must be made to ensure that the carer is positioned behind the X-ray tube head, and if available they should be offered lead rubber protective aprons to protect them against backscatter coming from the patient.

There are a variety of means of preventing access to the controlled area by unauthorised persons:

- Automatic warnings outside the door. As soon as the mains supply to the X-ray machine is switched on, a light or sign is illuminated outside the surgery with the legend 'X-ray examination in progress. Do not enter.' Or similar.
- A permanent or removable side outside the surgery door with the legend 'X-ray examination in progress. Do not enter.' Removable signs must be appropriately placed and permanent ones unobstructed.

With either of these signs, it should also be that the surgery door is closed as in general people will take an open door as a sign that it is safe to enter.

- The final method would be for a person to stand in the doorway to physically prevent entry by unauthorised persons.

The last is probably the most often used method but is the least favoured by safety organisations. If this method is to be employed, it is essential that the doorway does *not* fall within the controlled area during the exposure in question.

Mains isolators

The mains isolator for the X-ray equipment must not be left switched on all day every day. Leaving the mains isolator switched on while radiographs are not being taken increases the risk of accidental exposures to other persons, staff or patients not undergoing X-ray examinations.

This is particularly the case where the exposure switch is positioned outside the surgery; children playing around or staff accidentally leaning on the exposure button could easily activate the machine, potentially giving any one in the room an unnecessary radiation dose.

Even where the exposure button is in the room, someone could accidentally activate the exposure button.

The rule to follow is that when an X-ray exposure is required, it should not be possible to initiate this exposure by operating one switch/button only. You must have to perform two actions to make the machine produce radiation.

Examples:

Mains on	Activate exposure button
Type in patient details	Activate exposure button
Orientate image receptor	Activate exposure button
Open key cupboard	Activate exposure button

These alternatives to switch on mains are in place because for some digital units it is advised that the mains supply is not switched off to avoid disruption to the software.

Each of the four examples given earlier fulfils the rule of performing two definite actions to make an exposure take place.

The second rule for the mains isolator is that it must be positioned immediately adjacent to the position that the operator occupies to make the exposure; if this is not possible, it must be very close by. The reason for this is that the operator must have immediate easy access to the isolator in case of accidents.

Remember the regulation on contingency plans: 'in case of accident switch off at the mains immediately'.

The delay in cutting the mains supply should be as short as possible relative to the exposure time. Exposure times of 0.12 of a second or less are common, so if the exposure fails to terminate and it takes the operator 0.5 of a second to realise and then another 1 s to reach the mains isolator, then patient will have had an additional 1.5 s of radiation exposure or more than ten times as much dose as the expected dose for the examination.

In general terms this means that if the operator makes the exposure while standing in the surgery, the isolator must not be outside. The opposite is also true; it doesn't matter how sure you are that you know where the switch is if you have to step through or reach round a doorway. There is going to be a considerable (in relation to the exposure time) delay in operating the switch.

The last of the major points relating to mains isolators is that it should be positioned in such a way that it will never be within the controlled area. This is to avoid a situation where any emergency would make it necessary for a member of staff to step into the controlled area potentially receiving a dose of radiation in order to switch off the mains supply.

Operator's position

It is essential that the operator is able to see both the control panel and the patient at the time of the exposure.

The control panel should be visible in order that the operator is aware that the exposure has taken place.

The patient must be visible so that if they should move immediately before the exposure takes place, the operator is able to abort the examination.

Local rules and radiation protection supervisors

Local rules

There must be written local rules for all controlled areas, and they must be relevant to the work carried out in that area.

This relevance to the work carried out means that the local rules must be specifically written for each controlled area. This is because if the risk assessment for that controlled area has identified any specific hazard (such as wall that does not provide an adequate

LEGISLATION

barrier), the local rules in their standard operating procedures may say, 'Never direct the beam towards that wall.'

The local rules must be brought to the attention of those persons likely to be performing work in that room. This does not mean that the rules must be on display and only that staff are aware of the rules. There would not be time for anyone to read the local rules either before or during an examination.

Specific important details of potential hazards and the methods that should be employed to avoid harm to persons (standard operating instructions, schemes of work) should be displayed.

Radiation protection supervisors

One or more RPS must be appointed; the appointment must be made in writing, and they must have sufficient knowledge and authority to perform that tasks required of them.

The supervisor(s) is responsible for ensuring that all persons work within the regulations, schemes of work and local rules at all times.

This obviously means that they must be on the premises for the majority of the working week as it is impossible to supervise someone from 2 or 3 miles away.

Duties of manufacturers

Manufacturers are required to design and construct equipment so that it restricts as far as reasonably practicable all exposures to ionising radiation.

As part of this requirement, installation of equipment must include a critical examination that ensures that:

All safety and warning features are working properly.
Persons are adequately protected from ionising radiation.
They consult with the RPA on the required extent of testing.
The employer is given information on the use of the equipment and the required regular testing and maintenance.

A full report of the critical test and a critical examination certificate should be provided. The report will cover all working features of the equipment such as is the kV, mA and exposure time accurate, is the filtration, diameter of the exit beam adequate, etc.?

The purpose of this test and report is to demonstrate that the equipment is safe to be used.

The requirement for installers to give information on proper use is to ensure that radiation equipment is not left in the hands of people who are not able to use it safely.

Equipment for medical use

Equipment for medical use does of course include dental X-ray equipment. For such equipment the employer must ensure the equipment is fit for its intended purpose; this includes design manufacture and installation. The equipment must be capable of restricting exposures to those undergoing medical exposures as far as is reasonably practicable.

There should be some method for informing those using the equipment of the quantity of radiation produced during the exposure.

The employer should put into place a suitable quality assurance programme to make sure the equipment continues to restrict exposure to reasonable levels.

LEGISLATION

The quality assurance programme must include the following:

- Critical Examination and Acceptance testing before the equipment is first used.
- Testing of equipment performance at regular intervals and after major maintenance. The specific requirement for dental X-ray equipment is that full tests must be carried out at intervals no greater than 3 years. There is however strong advice that some form of testing is carried out each year.
- Assessment at regular intervals of the dose delivered to patients.
- Regular checks must be made that are designed to prevent malfunction of the equipment that would result in excessive doses to patients or other persons.

All parts of these regulations are enacted into law within the United Kingdom, and any non-compliance could result in criminal charges.

LEGISLATION

Chapter 11

Legislation: Ionising Radiation (Medical Exposures) Regulations 2000 (IR(ME)R 2000), Statutory Instrument 1059

Whereas IRR1999 is not designed to protect patients but workers and members of the public, IR(ME)R 2000 is specifically designed to provide the means to protect patients, hence the term 'medical exposures' in the title.

Patient in this case refers to someone undergoing an X-ray examination.

Within a dental practice patients sitting in the waiting room are not patients within the IR(ME)R definition, nor are those in the dental chair for a general inspection, scale and polish, extraction, etc.

For the majority of the time that a patient is in the practice, they are protected by IRR 1999 as a member of the public, not as a patient.

Once the decision is made to perform an X-ray examination, the status of the person changes to that of an IR(ME)R patient, and measures to restrict the medical exposure are implemented in the build-up to and during the completion of the examination.

The two major principles underpinning the restriction of medical exposures are 'justification for and optimisation of the radiation dose'.

The IR(ME)R regulations define four key roles:

1. Employer
2. Referrer
3. Practitioner
4. Operator

They also cover entitlement to act in any of these roles; this involves adequate training and the authority to act.

Quality assurance is also included within these regulations, but it is generally concerned with quality assurance of procedures.

Basic Guide to Dental Radiography, First Edition. Tim Reynolds.
© 2016 John Wiley & Sons, Ltd. Published 2016 by John Wiley & Sons, Ltd.

In general terms therefore IRR 1999 covers quality assurance of equipment (the things we use) and IR(ME)R, quality assurance of procedures (the things we do).

Medical exposures may be undertaken:

- As part of the patients' own diagnosis or treatment
- For the purposes of occupational health screening
- As part of a health screening programme
- For research where people are voluntarily participating for medical, biomedical, therapeutic or diagnostic purposes
- For medico-legal purposes

The first of these applies to dental practices and in rare cases the last two may apply.

DUTIES OF THE EMPLOYER

Although this section sets out the duties of the employer, it is important that everyone in the practice is aware that these requirements are met because if there is any non-compliance with these regulations, a portion of the responsibility rests with everyone involved in the radiographic process no matter how small their involvement is.

The employer shall:

- Ensure that there are written procedures in place for all medical exposures and that all practitioners and operators comply fully with their written procedures

This will include:

Procedures to identify the individual to be exposed
Identification of those entitled to act as referrer, practitioner or operator
Procedures for making enquiries of women of childbearing age
Procedures to ensure that quality assurance programmes are followed
Procedures for assessment of the patients' radiation dose
Procedures for the use of reference doses (this is a dose that you would not expect to exceed for 75% of persons having radiographs taken)

*It is not a requirement that women of childbearing age are asked if they are pregnant prior to dental radiographic examinations.

The advice states that 'There is no need to alter referral criteria in dental radiography based on the fact that the patient is pregnant'.

This means if the patient is pregnant and really needs an X-ray examination, you can go ahead and complete the examination.

If the decision is made that the treatment can be planned and implemented without the radiograph, the question must then be asked: 'Was it justified in the first place?'

If the routine is for the patients to be asked about their pregnancy status (many practices do make such an enquiry), there must be a written procedure.

If the policy is that the patient is not asked about potential pregnancy, there must again be a document stating this. It must be one or the other not individual choice.

- Put in place protocols for all standard radiological procedures with each piece of equipment

This will include items such as:

- Use of film holders (paralleling technique) unless it proves impossible to place them properly in the patients' mouth
- Appropriate film speed, sensor size, etc.
- Which exposure setting to use
- Establish:
  - Recommendations concerning referral criteria; (if outside referrals are accepted the referrer must be aware of the criteria and a list of approved referrers must be held)
  - Quality assurance programmes for standard operating procedures
  - Diagnostic reference dose levels for each examination with each item of equipment
- Take steps to ensure that all staff carrying out medical exposures shall:
  - Be adequately trained to perform the task
  - Undergo periodic continuing education and training
  - Competent to perform the specified tasks

DUTIES OF THE PRACTITIONER, OPERATOR AND REFERRER

In broad terms the practitioner is the person that justifies the individual medical exposure.

The operator is any person that carries out any practical aspect of the radiographic exposure; this would include loading the film holder, processing the film, etc. Any small practical part of the procedure makes a person an IR(ME)R operator:

- The first duty of both the practitioner and operator is to comply with all of the employers' written procedures.
- The practitioner justifies the exposure, ensuring that there is a clear clinical indication that the examination is necessary.
- The employer or practitioner can allocate any practical aspect of the procedure to any person or persons entitled to perform that particular practical task. (Entitled means those who have had adequate training and maintain their competence.)
- The operators themselves are responsible for any and all practical, radiography related tasks, that they perform.
- Referrers shall supply the practitioner with sufficient relevant information (e.g. previous diagnostic information or records) to enable the practitioner to assess the need for a medical exposure to take place and to assess that there will be net benefit for the patient (this means that the benefit of the radiation dose is greater than the hazard it produces).

In many cases within a dental practice, the dentist will be acting as referrer, practitioner and operator; this does not mean that the above does not apply. There must be written procedures as previously detailed, and those procedures must be followed.

In diagnostic facilities in hospitals, the referrer is a medical practitioner or other healthcare practitioner who is entitled. He/she examines the patient, and if they think an X-ray examination may be appropriate, they write a request card for the examination. This card includes all of the information relevant to the justification of the exposure (signs and symptoms, duration of symptoms and any significant features of the onset of the signs and symptoms) and finally the examination they think may be appropriate.

A radiologist or radiographer assesses the information given by looking at the risks and potential benefits of the exposure and makes a decision on whether to proceed with the examination or not.

This same procedure must be followed in a dental practice even if a single dental practitioner is acting in the roles of a referrer, practitioner and operator.

Where the practitioner is not also the operator, the practitioner must be certain that the person who will be initiating the exposure is competent to do so.

JUSTIFICATION OF MEDICAL EXPOSURES

Medical exposures cannot be carried out unless:

- It has been justified by the practitioner as showing sufficient benefit, taking into account:
  - The objectives of making the exposure (what will it be expected to show or to exclude)
  - The total health benefit to be derived by the individual to be exposed is assessed
  - The detriment (health problems) that the exposure may bring are assessed
  - The effectiveness and hazard of the X-ray examination has been assessed in relation to all alternative methods of obtaining the diagnostic information
- If the exposure is to be made for research purposes, it has been approved by a local research committee. For such exposures a dose constraint must also be formalised. This means a strict limit on the doses that will be used has been agreed.
- If it is an exposure for medico-legal reasons, it must fall within the employers' own written procedures for such exposures.

In considering justification of the exposure, the weight given to each of the factors must take into account the type of exposure:

Medico-legal.
Research.
Urgency of the exposure if the patient is a woman who is pregnant – this only applies if the practice policy is to question women of childbearing age as regards to their pregnancy status.

Optimisation

All medical exposures must be kept as low as reasonably practicable (ALARP), consistent with the intended purpose of that exposure.

This statement effectively says that the dose must be as low as possible as long as it does the job it was supposed to do. This means that if an exposure is made and the image does not include all of the information that it should have, the exposure must be repeated.

If an image does not include all of the information it was supposed to have shown and it is not repeated, it brings into question the original justification (i.e. if you could make do without some of the information, did you really need it in the first place?).

Reducing the dose to the patient is not a reason for failing to repeat an exposure that does not produce all of the diagnostic information it was supposed to deliver. In fact not repeating it means the dose has been unjustified, it was delivered for inadequate diagnostic return.

The regulations also state that the operator should select equipment and methods that ensure that each and every medical exposure meets the ALARP principle.

Although the employer will be responsible for the purchase of the major items of X-ray equipment, it is the responsibility of everyone to ensure it is used properly and in a manner that will ensure the dose is as low as practicable within the limits of its intended purpose.

This includes any additional or accessory items designed to reduce the dose or improve the quality of the image (e.g. film holders and rectangular collimators).

To fulfil this part of the regulatory requirements, operators must take into account:

Quality assurance measures
Efforts to assess patient dose
Adherence to diagnostic reference levels

A list of measures that may be used to reduce the dose to the patient can be found at the end of Chapter 9, 'Radiobiology'.

Employers should also ensure that the clinical outcome of every exposure is recorded in timely fashion; where the employer and practitioner are the same person (as may be the case in a dental practice), he or she is responsible for ensuring that the evaluation is properly recorded.

This literally means that if the result of an X-ray examination is not recorded, the procedure would be deemed to be not justified.

Factors relevant to the patient dose must also be recorded, so if the patient moved and the image repeated, it must be recorded as the diagnostic information would have been obtained at double the expected dose.

Clinical audit

Radiography and radiology must be the subject of clinical audit; this means that the quality of the images must be assessed as well as the quality of the diagnostic conclusions.

Grading of the quality of the image has been well publicised with the three grades 1, 2 and 3 representing:

1. A perfect radiograph with no errors of positioning, exposure or processing; 70% of the images produced should fall within this category.
2. There are errors in the image but it remains of diagnostic quality; 20% of images should fit this category.
3. There are errors which make the image non-diagnostic; no more than 10% of images should be in this category.

The radiological audit is more difficult, and it should involve peer group reviews of the diagnostic findings. This means a group of dental practitioners meeting to see if they all draw the same diagnostic conclusions from a number of radiographic images.

A brief summary of the requirements for justification and optimisation would be the following.

Justification

For a dose to be justified, enough clinical information must be gathered for a full assessment of the benefit to be derived by patient so that it can be weighed against the potential risks of the exposure.

This means that a full history must be taken and a clinical examination performed. The reason for taking the radiograph must be recorded before the exposure is made. The diagnostic result must be recorded soon after the image has been produced.

Optimisation

The best possible image must be produced at the lowest possible dose.

This means there must be quality assurance programmes covering the equipment used and the systems employed in producing the image.

The purchase of equipment able to meet the requirements of optimising the dose is essential.

If the first dose does not provide adequate diagnostic information, additional images must be produced in order to justify the original decision to deliver the dose to the patient.

There must be an ongoing audit of the results.

EXPERT ADVICE

The employer must employ a Medical Physics Expert (MPE) to give advice on matters such as:

Justification
Optimisation
Patient dosimetry
Quality assurance
Radiation protection

TRAINING

All those acting in the role of practitioner or operator must only do so if entitled to do so by having undergone adequate training and assessment in all practical aspects of radiography that they are required to perform.

The employer must keep an up-to-date record of all of those engaged to take medical exposures or to perform any practical aspect of any medical exposure.

This means that you should not carry out any part of the process of producing a radiograph unless:

You have been adequately trained.
There is detailed evidence of the training you have undertaken.
Your competence has been assessed.
Your name must be listed as a person competent to undertake that task.
You cannot undertake any task that is not listed as being within your competence.

> • Adequate training requirements for those initiating a medical exposure are detailed in Schedule 2 of the Ionising Radiations (Medical Exposures) Regulations 2000 and are reproduced in Appendix A to this text.

LEGISLATION

Chapter 12

Quality assurance

Quality assurance in radiography is not something that is 'a good idea if you have time', but is a legal requirement.

Broadly speaking IRR 1999 makes it a legal requirement for the practice to perform quality assurance testing on your equipment, and IR(ME)R 2000 requires that your procedures are quality assured.

The purpose of a fully integrated quality assurance programme is to identify faults in the imaging system before those faults have an adverse effect the radiograph of any patient.

In plain English this means the following:

If you use film, there should never be a situation where a periapical, bitewing or OPG comes out of the processor and you say, 'it's low density; the developer needs changing'. The programme should have identified a regular chemical change protocol that prevents films being processed with chemicals that are exhausted.

If you use digital phosphor plates, you should never view a patient's radiograph and think, 'That sensor has a lot of artefacts; it needs replacing'. This should have been decided before it was used on the patient.

Many people use the two terms quality assurance and quality control in the same way and interchange the two.

Quality assurance however is about overriding principles:

The desire to produce high-quality results
The setting of appropriate standards
Putting into place measures that ensure the standards are met
Assessing the outcomes (quality audit)
Promoting behavioural changes in staff where necessary

Quality control is about the things that are done to ensure the quality of the output, for example:

Ensuring film is stored in ideal or close to ideal conditions
Checking if film holders are in good condition before using them

Basic Guide to Dental Radiography, First Edition. Tim Reynolds.
© 2016 John Wiley & Sons, Ltd. Published 2016 by John Wiley & Sons, Ltd.

Making sure operators are using film holders whenever possible
Processor or sensor stepped-wedge tests are being performed
X-ray equipment tests

None of this can be left to the individual to perform as and when they think about it. The procedures must be written down in detail, the personnel responsible should be identified and properly trained to carry out all actions, there must be a schedule for all testing, and there must be checks that all of these scheduled procedures are carried out.

Included in this quality system will be:

X-ray equipment
Image receptors, film, phosphor plates or sensors
Accessory equipment:
  Film holders
  Cassettes
  Processing equipment
  Darkroom (if you still have one)
Working procedures
Staff training and updating
Audit of results, radiographic (how good was the image) and radiological (how accurate
  was the reading of the radiograph)

In trying to set out the requirements of an integrated quality assurance programme, there is some difficulty in knowing where to start and what order to follow. There is always the temptation to look at the big items first, those that have major impacts on image quality and the patient's radiation dose. That approach however implies that some items may be more important than others where in fact all play an equal part in achieving the aim of producing good diagnostic quality images at low radiation doses.

In order to overcome this difficulty, we shall try to follow a logical path starting with the things we do before the patient arrives following through to what must be done after the patient has left the practice.

STAFF TRAINING

We have already discussed this in Chapters 10 and 11: in Chapter 10 we saw the need for all staff to have received relevant training in the safe use of ionising radiation, and in Chapter 11 we saw the requirement for training staff to carry out any specific task related to radiography.

In each case there should be a record of the training undertaken. This record should be in sufficient detail so that anyone wishing to assess the competence of staff to perform any task can make reference to the training record and check to ensure that it meets any formal requirement, for example, that set out in Schedule 2 of IR(ME)R 2000 (adequate training for practitioners and operators).

In addition to the detail of the training received, there should be records of any examination of knowledge and also records of practical assessments of competence.

QUALITY ASSURANCE

There will also be records of the update training that has been completed and a schedule of future attendance.

In relation to update training, remember that 5% of your CPD every 5 years must be in radiology/radiography-related topics and at least 5 h of this must be verifiable. This requirement extends to all DCPs, even if they have no direct involvement in the radiographic process.

FILM STORAGE

This is an item that many tend to ignore taking the view that any cupboard will do.

Not too many years ago I was asked to look into the cause of a series of fogged, low-contrast poorly detailed radiographs that the practice could not solve.

Not being able to solve the puzzle on the telephone, I went along to have a look.

I found that their film was stored in a cupboard that contained pipes for the hot water system, not just for the taps but also the heating, so they were hot for as long as the heating was switched on. The cupboard was small and enclosed so there could be considerable heat build-up. The actual temperature in the cupboard was, on the day 31°C.

The cause of the poor-quality images was heat fogging of the film prior to its use.

Ideal film storage conditions

Temperature. Range 10–24°C (beware if you store it in the fridge). Most fridges operate below 10°C, and storing film in them will affect its response to radiation exposure.

Humidity. Range 30–50%. Most people know that films should not be stored in conditions that are too damp, but not many realise that they can also be stored in conditions that are too dry.

Radiation. Yes, this would seem to be common sense not to store film where it could be exposed to ionising radiation; however many do not realise that the film does not have to be exposed to enough radiation to produce an increase in density in order to affect the final image. If a film emulsion is exposed to a very small radiation dose, it may not cause a visible increase in density on processing. That initial exposure however sensitises the film, and it will react much more than it should to any subsequent exposure. This would mean that producing a radiograph with your standard exposure factors would result in an image with higher than intended density. There would also be reduced contrast and the diagnostic information would be degraded. The film store should therefore be well away from any potential source of ionising radiation.

Storage position. Film should not be stacked flat; it is usually the OPG film that is affected by this type of poor storage. It seems quite natural to store intra-oral film in the correct way because of the shape of the box (Figure 12.1a).

Although the edges of a box are quite strong, the centre is not. As you will know (if you have handled one), a box of OPG film has considerable weight. The result of stacking film is considerable downward pressure through the middle of the boxes onto the middle of the film (Figure 12.1b). This pressure can cause direct pressure artefacts, or it may change the films sensitivity to future exposure.

Chemical contamination. Exposure to chemical fumes prior to making the diagnostic exposure could, depending on the chemical, increase or decrease the reaction to ionising radiation; in either case the density, contrast and overall quality of the image will be affected.

QUALITY ASSURANCE

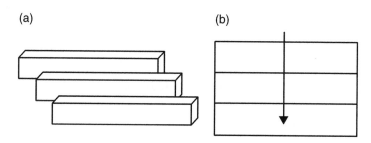

Figure 12.1 (a) Correct film storage position of boxes side by side. (b) Incorrect stacking of boxes

Stock rotation. Avoid the temptation to place new film into the first available space; the new film should be placed in a position that clearly identifies it as new stock so that the older film will be used first. If this system is not followed and new film is used first and an old box is suddenly discovered at the back of the cupboard, the temptation is to use it as it has been paid for. Avoid this temptation; depending on exactly how long it has been there, you may be producing severely substandard radiographs.

Remember storing films incorrectly may result in the patient's radiograph being reduced in diagnostic quality and in extreme cases could result in a repeat examination being necessary with the patient's radiation dose being doubled.

The rules on correct storage do not just apply to film.

Digital imaging phosphor plates must:

Not be subjected to direct pressure
Be kept away from extremes of temperature
Not be bent or creased
Not be placed on or moved along hard surfaces that may scratch the imaging area
Kept away from sources of radiation
Not be subjected to very high or very low humidity conditions

Charge coupled devices

Charge-coupled devices and wireless sensors are also subject to the conditions outlined previously for phosphor plates but in addition they must not be subjected to physical blow such as dropping them. There are, remember, small electrical components inside that could be broken or misaligned by sudden impacts.

Anyone handling any of these image receptors for any purpose must have received training in their proper handling and storage because mishandling, as explained earlier, could result in poor image quality or increased doses to patients.

FILM HOLDERS

When discussing quality assurance in dental radiography, the first thing to say about film holders is to use them whenever possible; they do, when used properly, produce a much better image than can be obtained with the bisecting angle technique.

Although the film holder looks to be a fairly simple item of equipment, what could go wrong with it? You should make certain checks before using one.

QUALITY ASSURANCE

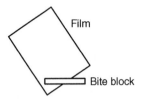

Figure 12.2 Film rotated in film holder

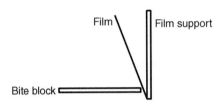

Figure 12.3 Film not properly supported in film holder

Is the film supported firmly? It must not be free to rotate once it is positioned in the holder (Figure 12.2).

If the film can move easily into a position like this within the holder, it may do so as the patient closes their mouth to bite on the block, and if the operator does not notice, some diagnostic information may be lost and a repeat examination may be necessary (Figure 12.2).

If the film is able to fall into this position (Figure 12.3), it will not maintain the essential relationship of being parallel to the tooth. If an image of the upper teeth were being taken in this illustration, the result would be distortion of the roots of the teeth.

If the film holder is of a type where the bite block and the film support can be removed from the main supporting arm, make sure the connection is secure before loading. If the bite block and holder come adrift from the arm as the patient closes their mouth, you may miss some vital information or have to repeat the examination.

Yes, the film holder is a simple device but you cannot leave it out of your quality assurance programme; it is just as capable of spoiling an image and making a second radiation dose necessary as your X-ray equipment and in fact is much more likely to do so.

CASSETTES

If you are still using film and cassettes for OPG or lateral cephalometry examinations, you will need to make certain checks on the cassette.

Is the cassette light tight?
Light tight cassette test
   To check this, load a film into the cassette and run an anglepoise lamp or bright torch round all of the edges. Process the film in the normal way and look for high-density (black) areas around the edge of the film. If there are black areas, the cassette has allowed the light to leak in. Light leakage of this type will reduce the quality of any image taken with that particular cassette.

QUALITY ASSURANCE

Are the screens in good condition?

Intensifying screen visual inspection

A simple visual check will tell you if there are any scratches or dents on the screen surface. These small defects are often more easily seen if you look at the cassette from the side, looking across the surface rather than directly at it. If the screens are dirty, they can be gently cleaned with a dust and lint-free cloth and the cleaning fluid recommended by the manufacturers. Soap and water should not be used, and even very mild nylon abrasive materials (kitchen pan scouring pad) will damage the surface.

Is the reactivity of the screen still at its optimum level?

Intensifying screen sensitivity

This simply means that the screen still produces the same density and contrast for a particular exposure as it did when it was new.

It is possible to test this with a large stepped wedge, if the exposure can be guaranteed as being identical and if the processor is also working at exactly the same level as when the last test was done.

As the X-ray machines and processor are part of your quality assurance programme, these items should be working at their optimum levels.

It is however much more reasonable to follow the manufacturers' guidelines. After a period of time or following a certain number of exposures, the performance of intensifying screen will fall off. In the literature provided with your screens, there will almost certainly be a section advising that screens are changed after either a period of time or after a specific number of exposures.

Follow this advice; remember you have a legal obligation to produce the best possible image. Using screens beyond their useful life will reduce image quality.

The manufacturers know the limitations of their equipment.

Is there good contact between the screens and the film?

Screen/film contact test

Poor contact between the screens and the film will increase the lateral spread of the light produced by the screens and will reduce the resolution of the image (there will be a loss of fine detail).

In extreme cases you will be able to assess this simply by applying light pressure to the lid of the cassette; if it moves up and down, the clips and/or hinges need adjusting or the cassette should be discarded.

We should say at this point that the cassette should never get to this level of disrepair; the fault should be found much earlier than this. It is almost certain that if you look at the latest patient images and compare them with those taken earlier in the cassettes' life, you will see a difference in the fine detail of the image.

Where the poor contact is not so obvious, there are specific test that can be carried out:

The most accurate method of assessing screen film contact is to place a perfectly flat fine wire mesh on top of the cassette and take a radiograph of it.

The wire of the mesh should be of around 1 mm and the spaces 2 mm. Care must be taken that the exposure is correct, particularly that the kV is not too high or the mesh will be penetrated, and even if the contact is good, the result will look poor.

If the screen film contact is good, the image of the mesh will have well-defined (sharp) areas; if the contact is poor, the image of the mesh will be blurred (on initial inspection there might be the appearance of different densities in some areas of the image).

If screen film contact is poor, it must be rectified as poor contact will reduce the amount of fine detail seen in the image and the diagnostic quality will be reduced.

An alternative for the wire mesh is to place something with a fine pattern into the cassette and then make an image using a very low exposure. The pattern must consist of fine areas of light and dark so that the light produced by the intensifying screens will pass easily through some parts and not others.

The problem with this second method is that the presence of the test object in the cassette will disguise the poor contact if it is slight because the space between the film and screen is effectively filled up by the object.

FILM PROCESSORS

It is of vital importance that those using film processors do all that they can to ensure that the machine is working at its optimum level at all times.

The processor is probably the single most common cause of poor radiographic results and repeat exposures.

Cleaning

One of the most important parts of ensuring no processor faults occur is to follow a regular cleaning routine; this usually goes along with the changing of the chemicals.

All of the roller racks and the tanks must be cleaned, strictly following the manufacturer's recommendations. No abrasive pads should be used or chemicals that are not recommended by the manufacturer.

Failure to clean the processor may result in gelatine marks on the image; these will be dark marks that look almost as if small pellets of grey black mud have been thrown at it.

Always take great care when replacing the roller racks, and make sure they go back into the correct position and are seated properly. If they are not seated properly, the guides for the film will be misaligned; if this is the case, films may become jammed in the processor, the image spoiled and an additional exposure to the patient required.

Temperature

Temperature is critical to the correct function of both developer and fixer; the processor is held at its optimum temperature by a heater and a thermostat. Modern processors have sensors and warning devices that tell you if the temperature is either too high or too low.

Older processors may not have these; where they do not, it is important that manual checks on temperature are made at regular intervals.

Persons operating the processors should learn to recognise faults from the resulting changes in the images that they produce.

If the processor is working well but then the radiographs produced are becoming more and more high density and contrast is reduced, it is likely that the temperature is rising due to a failure of the thermostat.

The purpose of the thermostat is to cut off the heater when the correct temperature has been reached; when the thermostat is broken, the heater goes on working and the chemicals heat up, increasing their effective activity.

If however the processor is working well but the density of the radiographs starts to fall off, it is likely that it is the heater that is at fault and the temperature is falling, causing the activity of the chemicals to fall off.

CHEMICAL LEVELS

As with the working temperature, modern processors also have sensors that indicate when the chemical levels fall; again if there are no such sensor and warning, it is important to carry out manual checks on these levels.

Low levels in the chemicals will result in the film not being immersed in them for sufficient time, and the radiograph will be under-developed and/or under-fixed.

Low chemical levels are not a common problem; however they can occur because there is always a little of the chemical carried out of the tanks despite the fact that there are rollers at the crossover that squeeze the film like an old-fashioned clothes mangle.

Chemical activity

We have already seen that temperature and chemical levels can affect the quality of the radiographic image; they are unlikely to do so as long as routine checks are made.

With ready-mixed chemicals the old problem of chemicals mixed in practice being either too strong or too weak in concentration no longer exists.

However as the processor is used, the chemicals do become exhausted and their activity slowly falls off.

Routine checks must be made to ensure that the falloff in activity of the chemicals is identified and corrected before it has a chance to adversely affect the radiograph of any patient.

The check that must be made is regular stepped-wedge testing.

The stepped-wedge test is carried out for two reasons:

1. To plan regular chemical changes that will renew the activity of the developer and fixer activity before any image of a patient has been affected by exhausted chemicals
2. To check that the activity on any particular day is at its optimum level

There are a number of different styles of stepped wedge on the market.

Generally speaking, the greater the number of steps on the wedge, the greater the accuracy of the test.

It is also possible to purchase test strips that have been pre-exposed to a known intensity of light.

The advantage of the pre-exposed test strips is that the level of exposure is absolutely guaranteed and the only variable in the result is the processing.

The disadvantage is the cost when compared with the standard stepped wedge.

Although many people use them, I am not an advocate of the home-made stepped wedge. The construction with a tongue depressor and lead foil from X-ray film packs results in a crude insensitive instrument that may fail to show subtle changes in the system before a patients' image is affected.

With the stepped wedge that is exposed in the practice, we can never be sure that any variation in the result is entirely due to the processor rather than the X-ray machine that made the exposure.

The only way to be sure of this would be to use a meter to test the output of the machine prior to exposing the wedge.

This would require the additional expense of purchasing a radiation output test meter.

Having raised this question, it is essential to say that the output of modern X-ray equipment is very stable, and it is highly unlikely that there will be any variation in output of a magnitude that is going to affect a stepped-wedge image on any given day.

QUALITY ASSURANCE

A standard stepped wedge exposed in the practice is therefore perfectly adequate for the purpose of ensuring standardised processor performance.

To adequately test processor performance, the stepped-wedge test should be carried out immediately following the chemical change and after the new chemicals have reached their correct operating temperature.

The frequency of retesting then depends on the throughput of the film, and it is rarely necessary to test every day, but at least two or three times per week is advisable.

Remember when large numbers of films are processed, the chemicals become exhausted more quickly and the stepped-wedge test must be completed more frequently.

Performing the stepped-wedge test

Place the wedge directly on top of the film.

Bring the X-ray tube down over the wedge until the end of the cone touches the surface of the table. This ensures that the distance from the focus to the film is standardised, eliminating variations due to the inverse square law (Figure 12.4).

Select the exposure to be used and make a note of it for use on all future tests (using the same exposure factors on the same X-ray machine is essential).

These features should be part of your quality assurance standard procedures.

After the exposure process of the film, if it is the first one following the chemical change, the image becomes your processor quality standard.

All subsequent tests should be compared with this standard. Look at a step in the middle of the wedge image and compare its density with the original. If they are the same, the chemicals are fine.

If the new wedge image has lower density, the chemicals are exhausted and should be changed.

Setting up a stepped-wedge test

The resulting image will look something like this (Figure 12.5):

When viewing the latest image of a stepped wedge, it must be compared with not just the previous one but a series of images (Figure 12.6).

Some suggest that rather than changing the chemicals when the wedge image changes, you can top up with a little new developer and test again. If the activity is not back to the original, add more new developer and keep on doing this until new developer has been added to return to the optimum operating conditions (I would not endorse this).

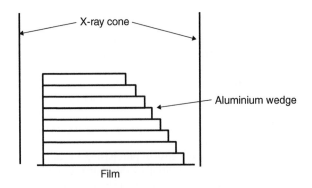

Figure 12.4 Correct positioning of film wedge and cone for a stepped-wedge test

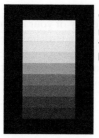

When the chemicals are new, the area of film where there is no wedge will look black

Figure 12.5 In a standard test: when the chemicals are new, there will be a completely black area surrounding the image of the wedge. This is because the wedge is smaller than a standard-sized film or phosphor plate, and X-rays will hit the film or plate directly all around the wedge, and it takes little exposure to make a film totally black when processed properly

Figure 12.6 A series of four wedge tests. It can be clearly seen that the first three tests, comparing each step with the same one in the neighbouring test show a consistent result. However in the fourth test, each step appears lighter than the corresponding test in each of the preceding three tests. The developer is underperforming because it has become exhausted

Topping up may have some success but only for a limited period and eventually the chemicals will need a complete change.

When the wedge test has been performed over a period, you will reach the point where you know that to maintain optimum processor performance, you need:

To add (X) ml of developer every (Y) days in order to maintain optimum activity (this can be continued up to the date of the complete change)
To have complete chemical change every 30 days or as specified by the manufacturers

The choice to use the stepped wedge or pre-exposed test strips or to top up or always go immediately to a complete chemical change is to be decided by practice (legal person).

However it must be kept in mind that topping up has limited effect particularly in the small dental tanks and will not be a long-term solution to the processing problem and is not recommended.

The performance of one or more of these tests and the employment of a programme for maintaining processor performance are legal requirement.

Remember the test is for processor activity and it does not and cannot test X-ray equipment output.

QUALITY ASSURANCE

DARKROOM TESTING

Not many dental practices now have a darkroom as most processors are usable in daylight conditions; if you do however still use a conventional darkroom there are some essential test to be carried out.

The simplest tests are purely visual.

Is the darkroom light tight? The human eye is very sensitive to light and it is the only
  equipment you need to test the light tight integrity of your darkroom.
Enter the darkroom and put off all of the lights (standard and safelighting).
Wait 1 min for the dark adaption of your sight to stabilise and then simply have a good
  look round the whole of the room to see if you can see any light leaking in.
Pay particular attention to areas around windows and doors.
Any leaks can be sealed with draft excluders of black tape.

Are the safelight filters in good condition?

Again a simple visual check is sufficient.
With the main lights out and safe lights on, make a close inspection of the safelight
to see if you can see any white light through small cracks or pinpricks in the coloured
filter.
If there are any areas of white light showing through, a new filter will be required; do not
try to repair it with bits of red or orange tape. This will almost certainly not be successful.

The final test requires a little more preparation and it is a test for the safe handling
time (this means how long can the film be exposed to the safelight conditions without
there being a noticeable increase in density).
This increase in density would be due to safelight fogging and would reduce the
contrast and fine detail seen on any image.

Setting up the safelight test

To perform this test you will need six coins or some similar object and a piece of thick
dark card large enough to cover the whole of an OPG film and also a watch with second
hand that you can see under safelight conditions.
  Lay the film on a work surface; with all of the lights out, then set out the coins at regular intervals on the film and completely cover with the card.
  Put on the safelight, pull the card back far enough to uncover the first coin and time
1 minute; then uncover the second coin, time another minute and uncover the third coin
and continue until the last coin has been uncovered for a minute and then process the film.
  The first coin will have been exposed to safelight for 6 min and the last one for 1 min
Figure 12.7.
  You will almost certainly be able to see the outline of the coins exposed for the greatest length of time. If you cannot see any outline of the coins exposed for 1 and 2 min, then
the safelight is fine (it should not be the case that any film you are processing is exposed
to direct safelight for more than 2 min).
  If you can see an outline of the coin exposed for only 1 min, there is probably some
fault with the safelight; you can do a further test with six coins again but uncover them
at 10 s intervals. This will tell you at what point in that first minute the increase in density
became detectable.
  At the end of the test, the coin in box A will have been exposed for 6 min, B for 5 min,
etc. The ideal result on processing the film would be that no outline of any coin is shown.
This is however unlikely, but if coin E that will have been exposed for only 2 min is visible
but F is not, we can accept that the safelights are fine. It will mean that the film will not
become fogged until over 1 min of exposure to the safelight. With good working practices, it is unlikely that the film will be exposed for a time greater than 1 min.
  If however the coin in position F (Figure 12.7) exposed for 1 minute is visible, we need
to repeat the test to see at what point in the minute the coin becomes visible. We do this

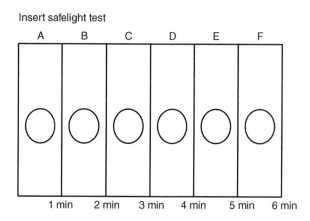

Figure 12.7 Safelight coin test preparation (A) exposed for 6 minutes (F) for 1 minute

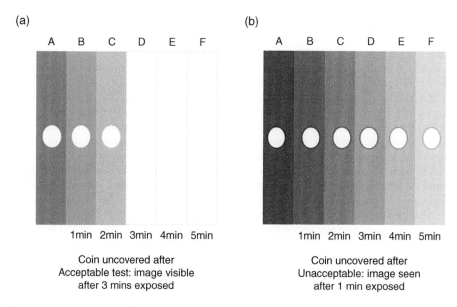

Figure 12.8 (a) Acceptable coin test result. (b) Unacceptable coin test result

by again placing six coins and revealing the next one in line at 10 s intervals. So the maximum exposure is 1 min and the least is 10 s.

Standard test with coins uncovered at 1 min interval
In the case of Figure 12.8b where the safe handling time is 1 min or less:

Carefully check the condition of the filters.
Check that it is the correct filter (is it compatible with your film sensitivity?).
Check distance from the safelight to the work surface.
Check the wattage of the bulb in the safelight.

QUALITY ASSURANCE

X-RAY EQUIPMENT QUALITY ASSURANCE

The radiation-producing X-ray equipment in your practice is tested before it is used on patients (preclinical critical examination), and it is then given a full test of performance every 3 years in accordance with IRR 1999.

It is further advised that interim checks should be made every year in an effort to ensure that radiographs can produce the required quality and within the reference dose of the practice.

These tests will ensure safe operation in terms of all of the major systems of the equipment; there are however a number of checks that should be carried out on a weekly basis by those members of staff who will be using the equipment.

The routine checks to be carried out are mainly visual inspections.

Physical checks

Where the unit is mounted on a wall, check that the fixing bolts have not come loose, there have been incidents in which the whole unit has fallen off the wall.

Check the opposite end of the arm at the point where the X-ray tube head joins the arm. Do these attachments seem secure? Again there have been incidents in which the tube head has fallen from the mounting. If this happens and the heavy tube head falls onto the patient, it may have serious consequences, for the patient or indeed the practice if there is a health and safety investigation.

Extend the supporting arms and check to see if the tube head will remain in position for each of the radiographic techniques you will be performing with this particular unit.

Remember that the counterbalances tend to work best when the arms are extended more fully. If the tube head does not remain in the required position, one or more of the joints may need tightening, and this should be a task left to an engineer.

The opposite can also be true: the tube head at some point becomes stiff and difficult to move. Where this is the case the mounting arm joints may need to be slackened off slightly; using a machine in this condition could result in injury to the patient.

Imagine the tube head is positioned close to the patient and then becomes stiff; you continue to apply pressure to position it correctly and it suddenly releases and bangs the patient in the face.

There is no defence in your favour as you were performing radiography with equipment that at the time was not fit for purpose.

Electrical safety

Electrical safety checks will be part of the formal checks made and reported on periodically by the engineers looking after your equipment; there are however additional simple checks that should be made on a regular basis.

Modern X-ray equipment has few, if any, exposed electrical cables. Where cables are visible, check on a regular basis to make sure that the insulating material is in good condition, not split or worn away by friction.

Also check the ends of the cables where the connections are made; these are the points that are subjected to most mechanical stress and where problems are most likely to be seen.

Where cable problems are apparent, an engineer must be consulted.

Check that the mineral oil is not leaking from the tube head; it will be a very light thin oil. Don't get confused by grease that the engineer may have used when refitting a cone/collimator. Leaking oil will be most often seen following an exposure or series of exposures; it is seen at this time because the oil gets hot and expands, pressure inside the tube head increases and oil is forced through any small fault in the sealing of the tube head.

The mineral oil provides electrical insulation so as more of it leaks out there is a greater chance of the 60–70 kV arcing across the tube housing and giving the patient a large electric shock.

The oil also provides part of the inherent filtration of the X-ray tube and housing; as more and more oil is lost, the filtration effect is reduced and more low-energy radiation will exit the X-ray tube, increasing the absorbed dose to the patient in terms of mGy/cm^2.

Radiation safety

There is really not very much you can do in-house to ensure equipment is performing properly in terms of radiation safety; this very much falls within the remit of the engineers performing the test for you.

You must however make sure that all safety controls and warning devices are working at all times.

In addition to this, if your X-ray tube housing is metal, check it regularly for dents. A dented tube housing could cause a crack in the lead lining, which in turn would allow radiation to leak through increasing doses to either patients or staff and possibly both.

Where a new dent is identified, place an intra-oral film or sensor over the dent and make an exposure; if there is no line or spot of density on the image, then no radiation is leaking. Put the test image in the radiation protection file (dated) and then mark and date (the dent as checked). Check similarly if a modern plastic tube head has a crack in it's surface.

If there is density on the film, an engineer must be called.

QUALITY ASSURANCE

Chapter 13

Dental intra-oral paralleling techniques

In describing intra-oral techniques, we are going to concentrate on the use of film holders (extended cone paralleling technique) because:

This technique will produce a much more accurate diagnostic result. When performed properly it will (for all practical purposes) eliminate the common distortion faults found in intra-oral dental radiography.

The patients overall dose profile will be reduced because there will be a reduction in the number of times an examination must be repeated due to errors.

The accurate use of rectangular collimators is much more achievable because the holder assists with the lining up of the central ray.

The technique is reproducible; this means that no matter how many times a single operator produces an image of a tooth or how many operators image that tooth, the image will always be the same unless the condition of the patients anatomy has changes. This makes it the ideal technique for long-term follow-up radiographs.

There is no regulation that says it is illegal to take radiographs using the bisecting angle technique.

However, IR(ME)R requires that we produce the best possible image at the lowest possible dose; film holders and the paralleling technique are a major aid in achieving this aim.

The bisecting angle technique still has a place because it is sometimes impossible to adequately place a holder in position. This will particularly be the case where the patient has a shallow palate, narrow dental arch, recent trauma or surgery and in the case of some anatomical anomalies.

Patients that tend to gag can still be persuaded to accept a film holder if the technique is approached in the proper way.

One key to a successful placement of the film holder is to make sure it is in the correct position the first time and is not placed too close to the teeth where it can irritate the palate or parts of the lower sulcus.

The correct placement will be demonstrated later, but in general the aim is to utilise the full length of the bite block to place the film into an area of the mouth where there is sufficient room for the film to stand parallel to the teeth.

Basic Guide to Dental Radiography, First Edition. Tim Reynolds.
© 2016 John Wiley & Sons, Ltd. Published 2016 by John Wiley & Sons, Ltd.

If the patient is noted to have a strong gag reflex, there are a number of measures that can assist with film insertion:

Try distraction techniques such as the patient making small circles with one of their feet or touching their thumb to each finger in turn.
Film is in a waterproof packet and digital sensors in waterproof cross infection control sheath so either can be quickly passed under a running tap to moisten them. This will often prevent gagging as a gag often occurs because of the dry instrument being placed into the moist environment of the mouth.

In very pronounced cases the patient tapping repeatedly for around 15 s on the area just above the point of the chin can be very effective in reducing the gag reflex; it is an acupuncture pressure point.

PERFORMING THE EXAMINATION

When undertaking any radiographic examination, the aim must be to produce a high-quality image at the first attempt. In trying to achieve first time success, it is important that things are done, as far as possible, in exactly the same way each time.

This is what professional sports people are attempting to achieve when they practise for hour after hour, day after day.

In performing intra-oral radiography, the position of the patient's head does not make any difference to the appearance of the image as long as the film holder and X-ray tube cone are correctly lined up with each other. However if the head is always placed in the same position, the operator will get used to the way things look and will come to a point of competence where almost instinctively they know when things are correct.

A way of positioning the patient's head is to use a number of positioning planes (external skin markers) to make sure that each patient is placed in exactly the same position prior to the film holder being inserted into the mouth.

When the film holder is then positioned, for example, for an upper right six, the position will look just the same as the last time an upper right six was imaged.

The planes that we use for such positioning are:

The median sagittal plane
This is a line down the middle of the face dividing the body into equal left and right halves.
For intra-oral radiography the patient is seated erect with this line positioned vertically.

The upper positioning line
This line extends from the ala of the nose to the top of the tragus of the ear; it is parallel to the occlusal plane and is 2 cm above it.
The upper positioning line is placed horizontally for all paralleling techniques, that is, upper and lower periapicals, also for upper periapicals using the bisecting angle technique and for upper occlusals. The line is placed in a horizontal position to ensure that the occlusal plane is horizontal.

DENTAL INTRA-ORAL

The lower positioning line

    This line is from the canthus of the mouth (join between the upper and lower lip) to the tragus of the ear. This line is parallel to and 1 cm above the lower occlusal plane when the mouth is open.

    The lower positioning line is placed horizontally for lower periapicals taken with the bisecting angle technique and lower occlusals. The aim is to ensure that for these lower periapical and occlusal examinations, the lower occlusal plane is horizontal.

    The reason that we use these lines to position the occlusal plane is that once the mouth is closed you can't see the occlusal plane, so the external markers tell us when the occlusal plane is horizontal.

    Remember that perfectly good radiographic images can be produced without positioning the head as described previously as long as the film holder and film/sensor are accurately positioned and that the X-ray tube (central ray) is properly lined up with the holder.

    The positioning lines simply help to standardise the method used and the appearance of the film holder in place so that correct performance of the examination becomes one of those task you complete almost without thinking about it.

    The remainder of this chapter will address only the performance of the examination and the assessment of the image.

    We will not be discussing the reasons for undertaking the examinations, the clinical justifications or the radiological results as these subjects fall within the remit of radiological not radiographic texts.

    As an operator performing the task, it is not your responsibility to ensure that the clinical information is sufficient to justify the procedure; this responsibility lies with the practitioner.

    If however you know that any of the following is true:

- Patients are not being examined prior to the examination request.
- The reason for taking it is not recorded in the patient's notes.
- The results of radiographs are not recorded as soon as possible.

    You should not perform the examination as any of the aforementioned automatically means that the examination is not justified.

    Additionally, if you are not sure why the examination is being taken or the referral does not seem to match the patient's reason for attending, you should ask the practitioner for clarification. This is because as an operator, you should not initiate an exposure if you do not have a clear idea of the clinical justification.

INTRA-ORAL PARALLELING TECHNIQUES

You will remember when we discussed the geometry of imaging, we concluded that the most important consideration in presenting a good image is to keep the object (tooth) and the image recording plate (film or sensor) parallel to each other.

    To achieve this it is important that the film holder is placed carefully into a position where there is room in the mouth for the film/sensor to stand parallel to the tooth/teeth under examination. This statement was made on (page 128), but it is worth emphasising it once again.

DENTAL INTRA-ORAL

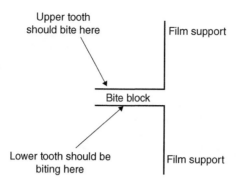

Figure 13.1 Correct position for teeth on bite block

It invariably means placing the film or sensor much further from the teeth than has become generally accepted (Figure 13.1).

The impulse (or instruction) to pull the film closer and closer to the teeth as the patient closes their mouth must be resisted.

General rule for positioning film holders

To understand the reason for maintaining large distance between the teeth under examination and the film, viewing the general anatomy of the oral cavity soon reveals the answer.

We need the film to be placed in a position in which there is adequate space for it to stand parallel to the teeth.

This means:

For the anterior teeth the film is placed towards the posterior portions of the mouth where the arch of the palate or floor of the mouth allows sufficient room for the film to stand. There will also be enough space between the left and right side of the dental arch for the film to adequately fit between them.

For the posterior teeth the film will be towards the centre of the mouth (median sagittal plane), again the position at which the arch of the palate or floor of the mouth allows sufficient space for the film to stand parallel to the teeth.

You will note that in Figure 13.1 the bite position for lower teeth is shown as slightly closer to the film than for the upper teeth; this is possible because there is more room around the flexible floor of the mouth than there tends to be the case in the palate.

THE FILM HOLDERS

There are many different film holders on the market and just two of them are shown in the following.

Any of those on the market will, used properly, produce excellent results; the emphasis here is on being used properly.

DENTAL INTRA-ORAL

(a)   (b)

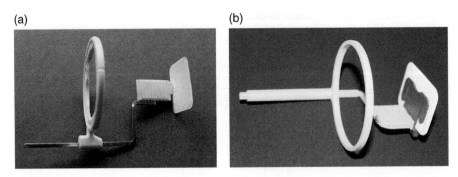

Figure 13.2 (a) Dentsply RINN posterior holder. Source: RINN product range reproduced with kind permission of Dentsply. (b) Kerr Super-Bite posterior holder. Source: Reproduced with kind permission of Kerr Dental

(a)   (b)

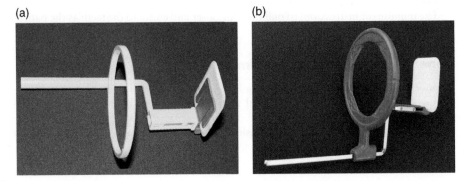

Figure 13.3 (a) Kerr Super-Bite anterior holder. Source: Reproduced with kind permission of Kerr Dental. (b) Dentsply RINN anterior holder. Source: RINN product range reproduced with kind permission of Dentsply

EXAMPLES OF FILM HOLDERS

Figures 13.2a and b are examples of holders used for the imaging of posterior teeth.

The holder shown in Figure 13.2a is currently set for images of the upper right; the short arm of the holder points to the patient's right and the film points up towards the ceiling.

Set up in this way, the holder can also be used to produce images of the lower left side.

The holder in Figure 13.2b is set up for the upper left; the short arm points to the patient's left and the film points up to the ceiling. Set up in this way, the holder can also be used to produce images of the lower right (Figure 13.3a and b).

The holder shown in Figure 13.3a is set up to produce radiographs of upper left or lower right anterior teeth. You will notice that the holder shown in Figure 13.3b has a straight arm with no 'L'-shaped bend, so it can be used on either side around the anterior teeth.

One feature you will notice immediately on picking up these holders is that the bite block is much longer on anterior holders than it is on the posterior ones. This is because when imaging anterior teeth, upper teeth in particular, a much larger distance is needed between the tooth and the film in order to maintain the essential, parallel, relationship.

ASSEMBLING THE FILM HOLDERS

It doesn't matter which particular manufacturers' film holders are used; the general rules for assembling them remain consistent.

Many people have difficulty with the assembly of film holders, but the few simple rules to remember are:

Think of yourself as the patient, so position the holder as if it is going into your own mouth. That means the long rod pointing away from your own face.
If you are imaging the left side, the short arm of the holder should point to your left, and for the right side, the short arm points to the right.
For upper teeth the film support points towards the ceiling; for lower teeth the film support points towards the floor. Following these simple rules will allow you to prepare a holder for any technique.

Remember that when a holder will fit for upper left, it will also fit for lower right, and upper right will fit lower left.

THE FILM

Dental radiography film has a small embossed blip in one corner. The blip is the anatomical marker; it tells us whether we are looking at teeth on the left or right side of the patient's mouth. If the standard placement of the blip is used, anyone can pick up the image and know which teeth they are looking at.

The correct placement of the blip for periapical radiography is that it should be towards the bite surface. This placement is easy to achieve for a periapical; we simply need to ensure that the blip is inserted first into the groove of the bite block.

If the blip is by the bite block, then it must also be by the biting surface of the teeth. To emphasise this point, the blip should never be by the apices of the teeth.

DENTAL INTRA-ORAL

- Figure 13.4a shows the position of the blip for upper periapical projections and Figure 13.4b for lower periapical. When in these positions, the blip is guaranteed to be at the crown (biting surface of the teeth.

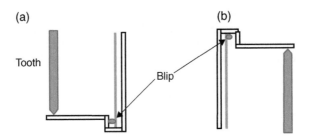

Figure 13.4 (a) Blip position upper teeth. (b) Blip position lower teeth

THE CENTRAL RAY

The central ray must pass through the ring of the holder to hit the film at right angles directly in its centre.

To make sure this will be the case:

Always look directly through the ring of the holder before use to ensure that the centre of the aiming ring is perfectly lined up with the centre of the film. If it is not you will need to reposition the ring.

It will now be correct but always recheck; you do not want to miss the majority of the area you were aiming for because you failed to make a simple check that takes less than a second.

PLACING THE HOLDERS INTO THE PATIENT'S MOUTH

No patient will open their mouth wide enough to simply put a film holder and film straight into it; not only are they reluctant but may have naturally limited opening. To overcome this it is advisable to start with the film in a horizontal position and rotate it towards a more vertical placement as it is gently moved towards the desired position, towards the back or middle of the mouth.

The movement required will be a rotation of the wrist.

The sequence of photographs in the following shows the stages of film holder insertion for upper anterior teeth.

UPPER ANTERIOR FILM HOLDER PLACEMENT

• Figure 13.5a–c shows the sequence for successful placement of an upper anterior film holder. Starting with the film horizontal gently rotate until it is parallel to the teeth, at the same time move the film towards the back of the mouth. Once the bite block is in contact with the upper teeth, the patient gently closes while the operator allows the holder to tip into the natural position with the film parallel to the teeth.

DENTAL INTRA-ORAL

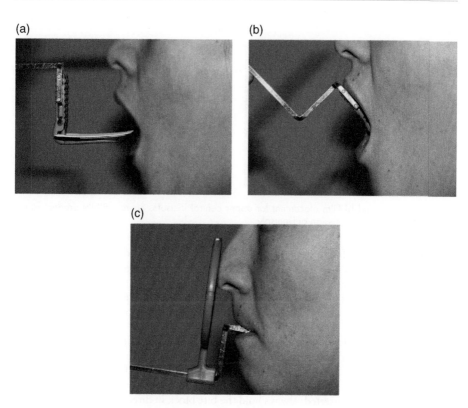

Figure 13.5 (a) Starting position, (b) mid insertion, (c) final position. Source: RINN product range reproduced with kind permission of Dentsply

The aim will be to get the bite block into a position where the tooth being examined is positioned centrally on the bite block. If two teeth are being examined, the interdental space between them will be in the centre of the block, and if three teeth are under examination, then the central one of the three would be in the middle of the block.

> • Here (Figure 13.6a and b), we see the position of the film holder prior to the patient closing their mouth when the upper central incisors are being examined. The interdental area (1-1) is directly in the middle of the bite block, and the film is placed well back in the palate, in this case just mesial of the upper 6. In some cases it will need to be even further back than this.

What we are trying to achieve here is for the centre of the area under examination to be positioned directly in the centre of image. When the main area of interest is in the middle of the film, then the best possible image will be obtained (you will recall this from the earlier discussions of imaging geometry).

As with all rules, there are exceptions; if the tooth being examined is at the back of the mouth, let's say lower right 7, then there is no point in placing the film such that the tooth

(a)   (b)

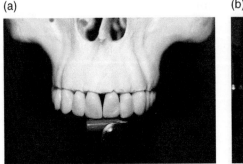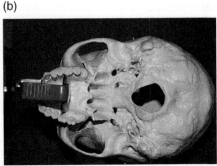

Figure 13.6 (a and b) Film placement for upper central incisors. Source: RINN product range reproduced with kind permission of Dentsply

is in the middle of the film. The reason we say this is, if the lower right 7 is the last standing molar and there is no 8, there is no point in irradiating a large area of tissue behind the LR7 where little or no diagnostic information can be gained.

This would mean not making the best use of the radiation dose (optimisation) in that all of the dose derived from the exposed area behind the LR7 is of little or no benefit to the patient.

In these circumstances it is much better to ensure that you include all of the LR7 and the alveolar margin immediately behind it and as much anterior anatomical detail as possible. In this way incidental diagnostic information may be picked up so that the dose has been optimised.

When the holder is inserted, always hold the bite block in direct contact with the teeth being examined and then support the holder gently while the patient closes their mouth; let the holder tip into the natural position parallel to the teeth.

The sequence of images at Figure 13.5, upper central incisors, note that the images show the bite block directly contacting the upper centrals prior to the patient closing their mouth.

The reason for this is; holding the bite block against the lower teeth tends to cause the operator to hold the arm of the holder in a horizontal position. In this position the film will not be parallel to the teeth, and when the patient closes the top of the film or sensor, it will dig into the patient's palate.

This will at best be very uncomfortable or possibly every painful. You will have lost the cooperation of the patient not just now but for future examinations.

It also allows the operator to make certain that the centre of the bite block is lined up with the centre of the area under examination.

As the patient closes on the block, **do not pull the film closer to the teeth**.

APPEARANCE OF AN IMAGE OF THE UPPER CENTRAL INCISORS

- The technique described previously for imaging upper central incisors would produce an image similar to this. Note the line indicating the central axis of the film coincides well with the interproximal space. The image is not perfect as the incisal edges of the teeth are almost on, rather than 3 mm above, the lower border because the vertical angle was directed too steeply downwards (Figure 13.7).

DENTAL INTRA-ORAL

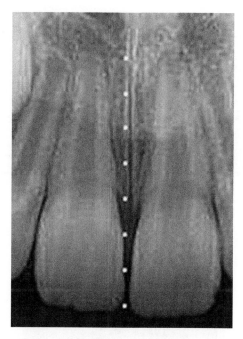

Figure 13.7 Image of upper central incisors.

This general pattern of insertion can be followed for any intra-oral examination.

The one additional problem you will encounter when imaging the lower teeth is the patient's tongue. The best advice is to ignore the tongue, not completely, just don't mention it to the patient. In general giving the patient any instruction concerning their tongue simply makes it active in the mouth and more difficult to deal with.

LOWER ANTERIOR FILM HOLDER PLACEMENT

To insert a holder for lower teeth, start with the film horizontal, just as we did for the upper teeth. Make sure the leading edge of the film is under the tongue, and then rotate and advance the film to the correct position. The tongue will be naturally pushed backwards out of the way.

- Figure 13.8a–c shows insertion of the film holder for lower central incisors. Starting with the film horizontal leading edge under the tongue, rotate the film until it is parallel with the teeth while easing it towards the back of the mouth. Central incisors should be centered to the bite-block. Support the film lightly against the lower incisors and ask the patient to close slowly and carefully. Let the holder tip into the natural and correct position.

The position we are aiming for prior to the patient closing onto the bite block is shown in the following (Figure 13.9a and b).

DENTAL INTRA-ORAL

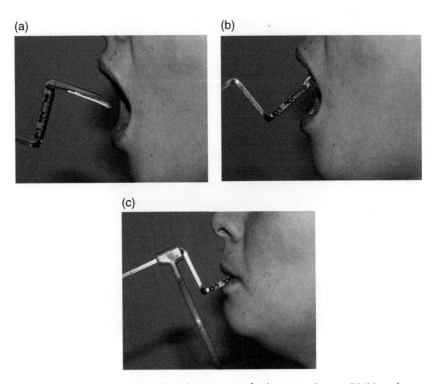

Figure 13.8 (a) Starting position, (b) mid insertion, (c) final position. Source: RINN product range reproduced with kind permission of Dentsply

- Figure 13.9a shows the bite block of the holder in contact with the lower central incisors with the interdental space lined up with the middle of the bite block. The film is positioned approximately at the lower six; in Figure 13.9b, you can clearly see the mandible would not be wide enough to accommodate the film further forward than this, and it would tend to twist no longer being parallel to the film.

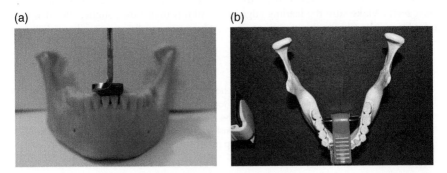

Figure 13.9 Film placement for lower central incisors. Source: RINN produce range reproduced with kind permission of Dentsply

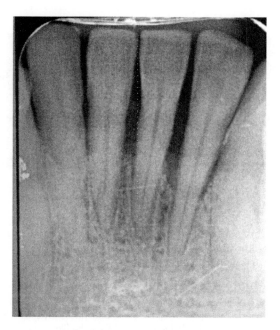

Figure 13.10 Image of lower central incisors

The image produced through the technique described previously would be similar to that shown in Figure 13.10.

- Note just as was required when imaging the upper central incisors, the central long axis of the film (dotted line) lies exactly on the interproximal area 1/1 (Figure 13.10).

UPPER POSTERIOR HOLDER PLACEMENT

This method of insertion, starting with the film horizontal, is exactly the same as it was for upper central incisors. It is however much more difficult to see where the bite block is in relation to the teeth, and it may be necessary to ease the lip and cheek out of the way. We need to do this to ensure that the middle of our area of interest is placed in the middle of the bite block and therefore in the middle of the film.

- Figure 13.11a shows the initial position of the holder. From this position rotate the holder until it is parallel with the teeth while moving towards the centre and back of the mouth. Figure 13.11b shows the final position of the holder.

Remember when inserting the holder the cheek should completely cover the bite block.

DENTAL INTRA-ORAL

(a)   (b)

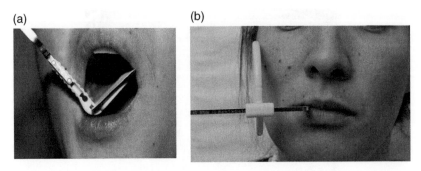

Figure 13.11 (a) Starting position, (b) final position. Source: RINN product range reproduced with kind permission of Dentsply

It may look difficult to achieve but the cheek is very flexible and the real objection that patients have is when the film digs into the palate; this can be prevented by ensuring that the film is placed well towards the median sagittal plane.

- Figure 13.12a shows the holder positioned for imaging of the upper right 5, 6, 7; the upper right 6 is placed in the middle of the bite block. This follows the rule that the centre of the area being examined should be in the middle of the film.
- Figure 13.12b shows the film in median sagittal plane where there is room for it to stand parallel to the teeth.
- Figure 13.12c shows the typical of radiograph produced.

(a)   (b)

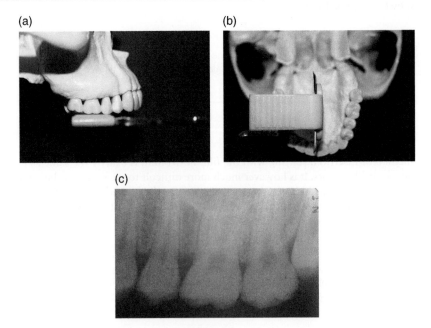

(c)

Figure 13.12 (a) Film placement (PA upper right 5, 6, 7), (b) PA upper right 5, 6, 7 and (c) shows the typical of radiograph produced. Source: RINN product range reproduced with kind permission of Dentsply

(a)   (b)

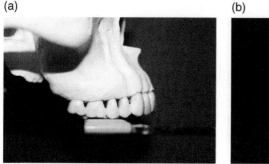
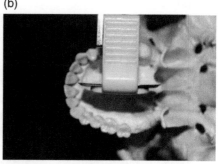

Figure 13.13 (a) Film placement (PA upper right 5, 6), (b) PA upper right 5, 6. Source: RINN product range reproduced with kind permission of Dentsply

- Here in Figure 13.13 we see the position of the holder when the main focus of the image is to be the upper right 5 and 6. The interdental space 5/6 is placed directly in the middle of the bite block.

LOWER POSTERIOR HOLDER PLACEMENT

Begin with the film in or near to a horizontal position; ask the patient to open their mouth and position the film so that the lower posterior corner is placed just under the tongue. The holder is then rotated to bring the film into a more vertical position while moving it towards the back of the mouth until the centre of the area being examined is lined up with the centre of the bite block. As with the technique for lower central incisors, the tongue will be pushed out the way as the film is advanced (Figure 13.14a–c).

- Figure 13.14a–c shows the stages of insertion of the film holder to for imaging of the lower posterior teeth. It is important to note that in Figure 13.14b the leading corner of the film is placed just below the tongue so that as the film is advanced it moves the tongue out of the way.

- For lower posterior teeth, we will be aiming to place the film parallel to the body of the mandible figure 13.15 and standing parallel to the teeth, and once again the centre of the area under examination should be located on the centre of the bite block. So for 5, 6, 7, the lower 6 would be in the centre of the block.

DENTAL INTRA-ORAL

(a)   (b)

(c)

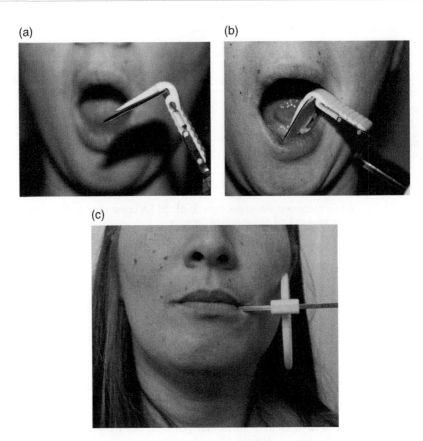

Figure 13.14 (a) Starting position, (b) mid insertion, (c) final position

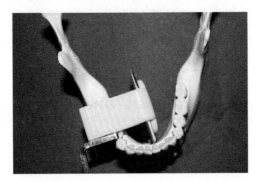

Figure 13.15 Film placement relative to lower molars/premolars. Source: RINN product range reproduced with kind permission of Dentsply

- An image of the lower 5, 6, 7 will look similar to this; (Figure 13.16) although the central axis of the film is not directly lined up with the centre of the lower 6, it is very close to being correct.

DENTAL INTRA-ORAL

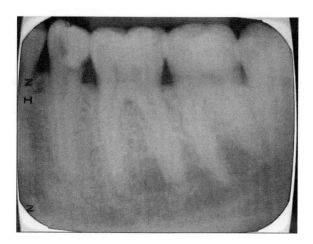

Figure 13.16 Image of PA lower 5, 6, 7

ASSESSMENT OF THE IMAGE

Having produced a radiograph, the next thing to do is to assess the image.

This assessment does not involve the diagnosis of the patient's condition; it is simply a check on the radiographic quality.

What we are doing here is looking to see if we have achieved:

The correct positioning of the film in the patient's mouth.
Correct alignment of the central ray of the X-ray beam.
Optimum processing (where appropriate) has been achieved.

It is essential that radiographs are always checked in this way before the diagnostic check is made, because if the radiograph has errors, those errors may make it difficult or impossible to make an accurate diagnosis.

If a system of checking is established and followed, it ensures that all factors will be taken into account for all images.

The following method for assessing radiographic quality works well, but it is only one way and it may be that the process currently used in your practice is perfectly serviceable.

Using the following headings will cover all of the factors that need to be assessed: Area, Projection, Density, Contrast, Sharpness, Artefacts and Grading.

RADIOGRAPHIC ASSESSMENT

Area

- Was the correct area included on the radiograph?
  Here we are initially checking if the correct teeth were included in the image and if we can see all of the area from the occlusal surface/incisal edge to around 4 mm above the apex.

DENTAL INTRA-ORAL

- Next, are we able to see any adjacent anatomy? This is important because symptoms are not always easy to locate, and a radiograph often reveals a problem close to but not exactly where it was expected.
- Was the centre of the area of interest centrally placed on the film? (except if it is the last molar)
- Is there a clear space of 3 mm between the incisal edge or occlusal surface and the edge of the film? (for a peri-apical radiograph)
  This is important because when a film or sensor is properly placed in the holder and the central ray is correctly aligned, there will be a 3 mm gap. So this can be used as an indication that other factors are incorrect.
- Is the orientation blip in the correct place?

Projection

Here we are assessing whether the central ray is correctly aligned, that is, was it perpendicular to the centre of the film?

- The simplest thing to check here is did we manage to direct the central ray to the middle of the film?
  Look all around the edge of the image, if there is an area that is completely clear (there has been no exposure), then the central ray was not directed to the middle of the film; there is 'cone cut'.
- Next we check to see if the central ray was perpendicular to the film. This involves the checking of two angles: the caudo-cranial (vertical) angle and the mesiodistal (lateral) angle; more familiar terms may be vertical and lateral angles.

- An X-ray beam directed along the black arrow would have a cranio-caudal angulation (head to feet) and the white arrow would be caudo-cranial (feet to head). Either of these would be incorrect, the central ray should follow the line of the holder. (Figure 13.17). The term vertical angle for this orientation of the beam is quite acceptable.

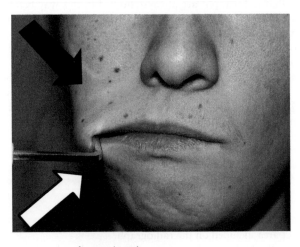

Figure 13.17 Demonstration of vertical angle

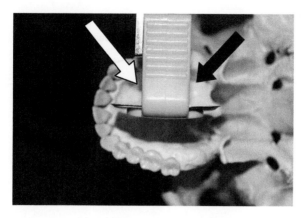

Figure 13.18 Demonstration of mesiodistal angle. Source: RINN product range reproduced with kind permission of Dentsply

- The white arrow shows a beam with a mesiodistal angulation (anterior to posterior), and the black arrow, a disto-mesial angle (posterior to anterior). It can be difficult to assess which of these two directions the beam is taking, and the assessment can use the single term lateral angle (Figure 13.18). The beam should follow the line of the holder not the arrows.

These angles form a very important part of the image assessment because if they are not correct, the accuracy of the subsequent diagnosis can be seriously damaged.

ASSESSMENT OF THE VERTICAL ANGLE

When the image is of the molar region, the vertical angle is relatively easy to assess because the bite surface is wide and has cusps on opposite sides; it is something like a dished surface.

- Figure 13.19 (a) shows how the X-ray beam passes through the molar cusps when the vertical angle is correct. When the images of the cusps appear at the same point on the film (they are superimposed), the crown is said to be in profile.
- In Figure 13.19b the vertical angle is incorrect, X-ray quanta originating from the same point will produce images of the cusps in different spots on the film; the cusps are not superimposed and the image will appear as if you are looking into the occlusal surface.

- Figure 13.20a shows the image produced when the vertical angle is assessed as correct when the crown is in profile; the two sets of cusps are superimposed.
- Figure 13.20b shows the appearance of the image when the angle is incorrect; we clearly see two separated sets of cusps, and we can imagine looking into the occlusal surface.

DENTAL INTRA-ORAL

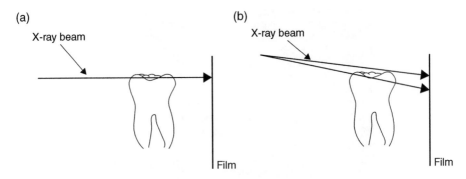

Figure 13.19 (a) Correct vertical angle. (b) Incorrect vertical angle

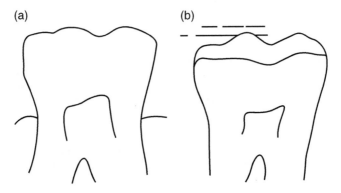

Figure 13.20 (a) Image correct vertical angle. (b) Image incorrect vertical angle

THE IMAGE

This method for assessing the vertical angle will not work when the images are incisors.

Because there is no broad occlusal surface, they are effectively a sharp blade. This means that the image of the incisal edge will be the same whatever we do with the vertical angle; it will present as a single sharp line.

- Figure 13.21a shows the X-ray beam with the vertical angle correct (90° to the film). When the film is loaded correctly into the holder, the image of the incisal edge will be 3 mm from the edge of the film.
- Figure 13.21b shows the situation when the vertical angle is incorrect. Depending on which direction the beam is angled; the incisal edge will be shown either more than or less than 3 mm from the edge of the film.

DENTAL INTRA-ORAL

(a)   (b)

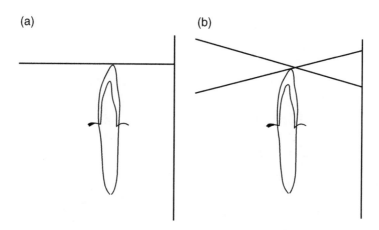

Figure 13.21 (a) Correct vertical and incisors. (b) Incorrect vertical angle and incisors

One of the checks we have to make when assessing the projection then is, does the image appear 3 mm from the edge of the film? This gap in itself is not important but it does tell us if the vertical angle is correct, that is, 90° to the film. If the angle is not correct, it can lead to a miss diagnosis because the size shape and position of features will change.

Where the distance from the bite surface of the tooth to the edge of the film is increased, the whole image is shifted, the result being that you may not demonstrate the 4 mm of tissue required at the apex of the tooth.

NB: The vertical angle cannot be assessed by looking for elongation or foreshortening. The paralleling technique performed correctly, that is, the film is parallel to the tooth, will for all practical purposes eliminate this type of distortion (see Figure 4.8a and b, page 48).

When assessing molars, it is not possible to demonstrate the crown in perfect profile because no person has perfectly symmetrical cusps. While this is true, this form of assessment provides a good general indicator. You can then, if you think the angle is incorrect, check the distance from the bite surface to the edge of the film for confirmation.

To demonstrate the importance of the vertical angle rather than draw a series of diagrams to prove a point, we will use some photographs of some small drinking glasses.

A roll of black paper has been placed in the glass to represent the pulp cavity of a molar and another piece placed on the rim to represent the area of caries.

- Figure 13.22a shows the relative positions of the pulp cavity and the caries when the vertical angle is correct (90° to the film).It is clear that the two features are entirely separate.
- Figure 13.22b shows what happens when the camera angle is changed to mimic a change in the vertical angle. The two features are continuous; is there involvement with the pulp cavity? Note, in Figure 13.22b, if you can see both rims of the glass, you are effectively looking into it in the same way that is seems we are looking into the occlusal surface, so you can tell that the vertical angle has changed.

(a)   (b)

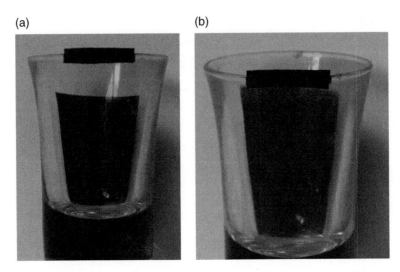

Figure 13.22 (a) Diagnosis, vertical angle correct. (b) Diagnosis, vertical angle incorrect

ASSESSING THE MESIODISTAL (LATERAL) ANGLE

Assessment of the mesiodistal angle remains consistent whether we are imaging incisors, premolars or molars. The assessment is based on the manner in which the beam passes between the teeth on its path to the film or sensor.

- In Figure 13.23 we can see how the image is formed when the mesiodistal angle is correct (black arrows). The X-ray photons pass directly between the teeth, and the interproximal spaces will be well demonstrated.
- When the angle is incorrect (white arrows), the photons do not have a clear path to the film; each one will make contact with parts of two different teeth. The result of this is overlapping of the images of the two teeth with no clear demonstration of the interproximal spaces.

- Figure 13.24a shows three small glasses representing 3 molars a piece of black paper representing an area of caries that shows clearly on the middle one of the three.
- Changing the camera angle (Figure 13.24b) to mimic changing the mesiodistal angle closes the gaps between the glasses. The area of caries is now smaller and we cannot tell if it is on the middle or left hand glass.

Having completed the assessment of the centring and orientation of the central ray, we then move on to assess the exposure and processing. This is achieved by looking at the density and contrast of the image.

DENTAL INTRA-ORAL

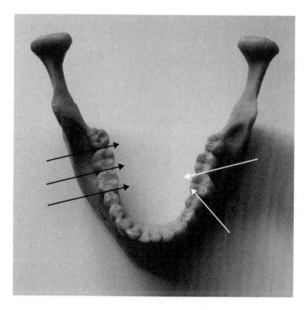

Figure 13.23 Demonstration of mesiodistal angle

(a)

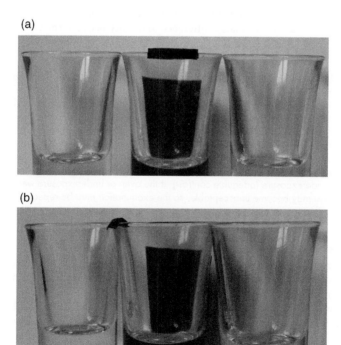

(b)

Figure 13.24 (a) Diagnosis lateral angle correct. (b) Diagnosis lateral angle incorrect

DENTAL INTRA-ORAL

DENSITY ASSESSMENT

This is basically the amount of blackness that we see on the image. There are two assessments to be made of density:

1. Check the directly exposed areas; these are the areas with the minimum amount of tissue lying between the X-ray tube and the film. This will be the most anterior part of the image and next to the bite surface of the teeth.

   This area should look close to black. If you are using film, a black directly exposed area only indicates that the film has been correctly processed and not correctly exposed, because when processing is optimum, it takes very little radiation to make the film go black.
2. To check the exposure on a periapical, you must also look at the apical areas to see if there has been sufficient exposure to make an adequate diagnosis of that area.

CONTRAST ASSESSMENT

Contrast is defined as the difference in density between adjacent areas.

What we are looking for is how clearly do the different tissues stand out from each other. Although there are many tissues that we need to see on a dental radiograph, the three areas we use to assess contrast are the pulp cavity, dentine and enamel. Ideally all three are visible, and there is a large difference in density between the three.

> • Figure 13.25 shows five boxes filled with different shades. If we take these shades as being the possible range of densities that may be demonstrated on a radiograph, we would wish pulp to show similar to box E, dentine box C and enamel box A. If we achieve this we can say pulp dentine and enamel are demonstrated and show a wide range of densities, and the contrast is good. As an image is overexposed or processed, the density scale will be compressed and moved towards the C, D and E end of the density scale. It will move the other way with under exposure or inadequate processing. The figure shows pulp, dentine and enamel still distinguishable from each other after over- or underexposure (adequate contrast). If the over- or underexposure were greater, the contrast may become unacceptable, so the examination must be repeated.

Figure 13.25 shows how the contrast of the image can vary.

When the pulp cavity has density E, dentine C and enamel A, we can see all of those tissues, and there is a wide density difference between them (they really stand out).

The contrast is good. When we overexpose or overdevelop (in the case of film), the pulp remains density E but dentine changes to D and enamel C. Although we can see the tissues, the density difference has closed and the contrast is only adequate. Further overexposure or development will make these tissues difficult to differentiate.

Underexposure or under development will also change contrast but in the opposite direction. Enamel is density A, dentine B and pulp C. The contrast is again reduced to just adequate; any further underexposure or development will again make the tissues difficult to differentiate.

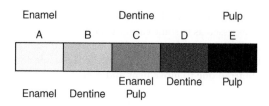

Figure 13.25 Demonstration of radiographic contrast

SHARPNESS ASSESSMENT

Sharpness refers to the fine detail in the subject and how well it is demonstrated in the image. When fine detail is not good radiographic texts tend to refer to unsharpness, though the word does not appear in the dictionary.

In a dental image the structures that are used to define this are the bony trabeculae (the fine honeycomb pattern in the bone), lamina dura (bony edges of the tooth socket) and the canal for the periodontal ligaments (Figure 13.26).

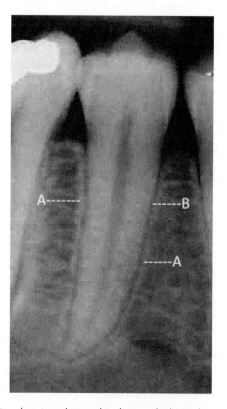

Figure 13.26 The lamina dura is a dense white line marked (A), the canal for the ligament is a dark line marked (B), and the bony trabeculae is a fine honeycomb appearance between the teeth. The bony trabecular pattern is probably the least reliable of the assessments as it is so variable. Source: Reproduced with permission of Katrina Hickenbotham

DENTAL INTRA-ORAL

Each of these structures should be clear and sharp on the image.

All three should be assessed as in some cases the bony trabeculae and lamina dura may look indistinct due to disease or reabsorption but the canal for the periodontal ligament is well defined. In such a situation looking only at the trabeculae and lamina the image could be assessed as blurred due to movement and repeated unnecessarily.

> • Note in Figure 13.26, the lamina dura is a dense white line, the canal for the ligament is a dark line and the bony trabeculae are in a fine honeycomb appearance.

ARTEFACTS

Artefacts are anything on the image that is not part of the patient and therefore should not be there. This means that none biological parts of the patient are not artefacts because they should be there. This excludes removable appliances.

When using film and processing artefacts, they would include:

- Gelatine marks from dirty rollers
- Scratches from poor handling
- Crimp marks (the dark marks that look like a thumbnail but are actually where the film has been allowed to bend under its own weight) common on OPG films
- Chemical marks

When using phosphor plates:

- Scratches from poor handling
- Light or dark pressure lines from bending
- Density marks from pre-exposure to radiation sources

When using sensors:

- Areas where no exposure seems to have taken place (filaments in the wire could be broken or detached).
- Changes in density not consistent with the image or pathology could be caused by damaged components in the sensor if it has been dropped.

If there are artefacts, do they interfere with the potential to make an accurate diagnosis? If so the examination may need to be repeated.

With all of the image recording systems, parts of the film holder may show if the vertical or lateral angles are incorrect.

For a film to be graded 1, all of the aforementioned factors must be assessed and they must all be correct. Remember a grade one will have no faults in positioning, exposure or processing.

If any of the above are incorrect the film immediately becomes grade 2, we then look again to see if it meets the diagnostic requirements (is it fit for purpose?) if not it must be repeated.

It is important to note here that making a decision between grade 1 and 2 is purely one of radiographic quality (it does not matter why the image was taken).

Deciding between grade 2 and 3 is radiological. Does the image provide the required information? If the answer here is no, then the image must be repeated or the exposure becomes a none justified one under IR(ME)R. (If a radiograph is taken for a particular reason but the information is not there and the decision is made not to repeat the examination, then why was it requested originally?).

Is saving the additional dose worth not getting the diagnostic information required for accurate assessment and treatment planning?

Any image must be assessed for radiographic accuracy before any radiological assessment is attempted. Factors that may affect diagnostic accuracy (as demonstrated in Figure 13.22b, page 148, and in Figure 13.24b on page 149, vertical and lateral angles) can then be properly taken into account.

BITEWING RADIOGRAPHS

The purpose of bitewing radiographs is to demonstrate the upper and lower teeth on a single film. The image will be produced to investigate interproximal caries and bone loss. The standard requirement would be to include the last interproximal space and at least 4 mm of upper and lower crestal bone.

In some cases the practitioner may request that you show the distal surface of the last standing molar rather than just the interproximal spaces.

Examples of bitewing film holders are shown in the following (Figure 13.27a, b and c).

Assembling the holders for bitewing radiography does not present the same problems of orientation sometimes experienced with periapical radiography. All of the examples shown previously in Figures 13.27a–c, set up as they are, could be used to produce an image of either the left or right side of the dentition.

The one difficulty that it presents is that of ensuring that the orientation blip is in the standard position for a bitewing radiograph.

The blip should be towards the mesial aspect of the image.

To place the blip correctly, it should be positioned so that it is close to the long arm of the film holder rather than on the free edge of the film. When in this position, the blip can be put into a mesial position for both left and right bitewing images. It will be opposite the upper teeth for one side and the lower teeth on the other.

BITEWING RADIOGRAPHS: PLACING THE HOLDER INTO THE MOUTH

The general rule for inserting film holders can be followed for bitewing radiographs and will be the same of those for periapicals.

Start with the film in a horizontal position; as soon as the leading edge is inside the mouth, start to turn the film into a vertical position at the same time it is moved towards the centre and back of the mouth.

DENTAL INTRA-ORAL

(a) (b)

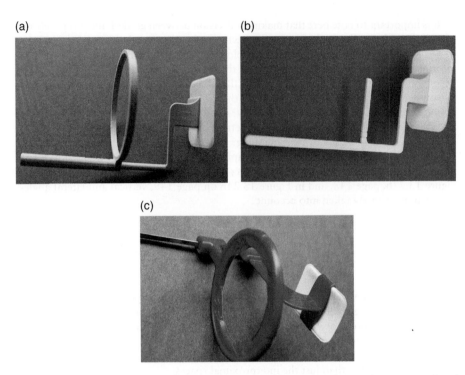

(c)

Figure 13.27 (a) Kerr Kwik-Bite ring and (b) Kerr Kwik-Bite index. Source: Images reproduced with kind permission of Kerr Dental. (c) Dentsply RINN bitewing holder. Source: RINN product range reproduced with kind permission of Dentsply

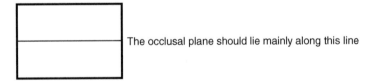 The occlusal plane should lie mainly along this line

Figure 13.28 Central axis for bitewing radiograph

The lower leading corner of the film should be the first part of the film to enter the mouth, and it should be placed just under the tongue so that the tongue is moved out of the way as the film is advanced.

It may be necessary to ease the cheek back to see where the posterior border of the film is to make sure that it will include the full area under investigation.

Insertion of the film tends to be easier for a bitewing than for periapical radiographs and presents less discomfort for patients because, obviously, only half of the film is in the lingual area and half in the palatal area rather than the whole of it being in one or the other as it would be for upper or lower periapical radiographs.

The aim is to place the film so that the posterior border includes the last interproximal space or the distal surface of the last molar (depending on the practitioners' request) and the central long axis of the film lies along the occlusal plane (Figure 13.28).

CENTAL LONG-AXIS POSITION FOR BITEWING RADIOGRAPHS

The following images show the start and final positions for a bitewing film holder.

> • As shown from the start position, the film is moved in three directions. Rotate the film until it is parallel with the teeth while simultaneously moving it towards the centre and back of the mouth (Figures 13.29 and 13.30a and b).

During the insertion of the film, it may be necessary to ease the patient's cheek to observe that the film is inserted into the correct position.

As with periapical imaging, do not pull the holder towards the cheek to position the film closer to the teeth during the time that the patient is closing their mouth.

Although this would seem to be a reasonable thing to do when looking at basic ideals of imaging geometry (Chapter 4). The large distance between the teeth and the film that will be evident when you position the film near the median sagittal plane has been compensated for by using the extended cone paralleling technique (Figure 4.7).

Once the film is positioned, the central ray can be lined up in the same way as would be the case for a periapical image. The end of the cone is placed in contact with the ring of the film holder; it is important that the whole of the rim of the cone is in contact. When this is achieved, it ensures that the central ray is perpendicular to the centre of the film.

When using the Hawe Kwik-Bite shown in Figure 13.24b, there is no ring to line up the end of the cone with so we need to find an alternative method.

The long arm of the holder must be lined up parallel with the edge of the cone in both the vertical and lateral directions. This will ensure that the central ray is perpendicular to the film.

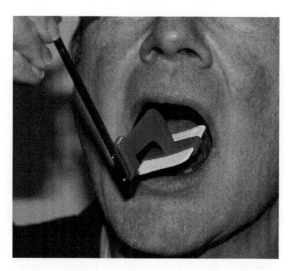

Figure 13.29 Inserting bitewing films. Source: RINN Product range reproduced with kind permission of Dentsply

DENTAL INTRA-ORAL

(a)   (b)

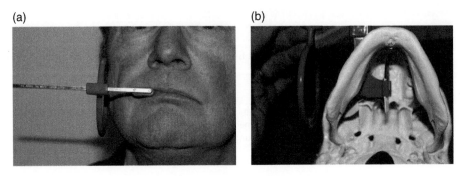

Figure 13.30 (a) Final film position for bitewing. (b) Film position for bitewing. Source: RINN Product range reproduced with kind permission of Dentsply

To ensure that the central ray is directed to the middle of the film, the end of the short guide arm must be positioned directly in the middle of the cone. To take into account the positioning of films/sensors of slightly different sizes, there are three potential positions for the edge of the cone:

1. In contact with the long arm of the holder
2. In contact with the first positioning notch
3. In contact with the second positioning notch

- The white lines on figure 13.31 show potential positions for the edge of the localising cone. They take into account the use of films of different sizes and the need to ensure that the centre of the cone is lined up with the centre of the film.

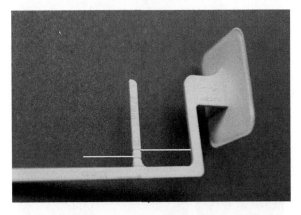

Figure 13.31 Kerr Kwik-Bite index, potential positions for the edge of the X-ray tube cone. Source: Image of the Kerr Kwik Bite Index reproduced with kind permission of Kerr Dental

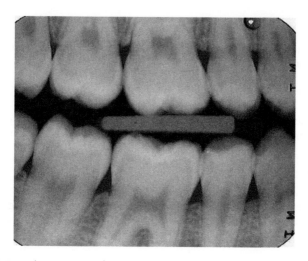

Figure 13.32 Typical appearance of a bitewing radiograph. Source: Reproduced with permission of Katrina Hickenbotham

- The positioning described for a bitewing radiograph will result in an image similar to this Figure 13.32: central axis largely coincident with the occlusal plane, last interproximal space shown, upper and lower crowns and sufficient bony detail.

ASSESSING THE BITEWING IMAGE

To produce a full assessment of a bitewing radiograph, the same system of checking should be used as that introduced for periapical images.

Area

Have you included the last interproximal space and as much mesial detail as possible (the first premolar should be shown)?

Is the central axis coincident with the occlusal plane (upper and lower crowns demonstrated equally and crestal bone seen)?

Is the blip demonstrated in a mesial position?

Projection

Was the central ray directed to the middle of the film (is there any cone cut)?

Was the vertical angle correct (are the crown in profile or can you see the occlusal surfaces (Figure 13.20a and b)?

Was the lateral angle correct? Are the interproximal spaces clear? Or is there overlap (Figure 13.24a and b, page 149)?

DENTAL INTRA-ORAL

Density

Is there sufficient density to make a diagnostic report for the crowns and the condition of the crestal bone?

Contrast

Are the pulp, dentine and enamel demonstrated? And is the density difference between them sufficient to adequately demonstrate all of those tissues and the margins between them?

Sharpness

Are the bony trabeculae, lamina dura and canal for the periodontal ligament demonstrated and well defined (sharp lines)?

Artefacts

Are there any features within the image that are not part of the patient and therefore should not be seen? If so are they interfering with the potential to make an accurate diagnosis?

Grading

Is the film perfect with no errors (grade 1), some errors but remains of diagnostic quality (grade 2) diagnostic or is it none diagnostic (grade 3) requiring a repeat examination?

DENTAL INTRA-ORAL

Chapter 14

Orthopantomography

This technique often referred to simply by the initials OPG or indeed as OPT or dentalpantomography (DPT). As the term OPG was the one originally used and is also the one common in general radiography, it is this terminology that we will continue to use for this text.

We have previously (Chapter 7) discussed the principals governing the production of an OPG image and do not need to cover them again at this point.

It is worth looking again at the advantages of the technique that was designed to replace older methods used to demonstrate the whole of the mandibular and maxillary dentition during a single examination.

Prior to the OPG full radiographic examination of these areas would require a sequence of 10–12 periapical radiographs or five occlusals.

The OPG:

- Is much less invasive for the patient
- Produces a significant reduction in radiation dose
- Makes assessment of the relative position of the teeth and their roots much more straightforward

  More diagnostic information of the surrounding area is available.
  There are of course some disadvantages:

- The full exposure requires that the patient is able to stand perfectly still for around 15 s. For some this can be quite difficult.
- There will always be some blurring of the examination area, and the amount of fine detail demonstrated will be less than other techniques.
- You need to purchase the specialist equipment to perform the technique.

PERFORMING THE EXAMINATION

Prior to the commencement of the examination, show the patient the movement that will take place so that they are not startled into moving during the exposure. This is particularly useful if the patient has not had an OPG previously.

Basic Guide to Dental Radiography, First Edition. Tim Reynolds.
© 2016 John Wiley & Sons, Ltd. Published 2016 by John Wiley & Sons, Ltd.

- Raise the machine to approximately the correct height for the patient.
- Ask the patient to step into the machine and place their chin onto the chin rest.
- Readjust the height of the machine so that the patient is not stretching or slumping but can stand comfortably. (If the patient is comfortable, they are much more likely to maintain the correct position throughout the exposure.)
- Ask them to take a firm grip of the handles. If the patient has broad shoulders, it helps to get them to cross their hands over (right hand to the left handle, left hand right handle). This reduces effective width of the patients' shoulders and prevents the machine making contact with them as it rotates.

Adjust the position of the patients' head so that

- They are biting upper and lower edge to edge in the grooves of the bite block. (This separates the upper and lower anterior teeth so that the overlap evident in the majority of patients' bite does not hide any detail. It also helps to ensure that both upper and lower anterior teeth remain within the focal trough.)
- The median sagittal plane is vertical.
- The inter-pupillary line is horizontal (so the head is not tilted left or right). This means that the X-ray beam will pass through left and right sides at the same angle relative to the teeth. If this is not correct, an uneven pattern of elongation and foreshortening may be seen making it difficult to make direct comparisons between left and right sides. This may reduce the effectiveness of the diagnosis.
- Frankfort plane is horizontal (Figure 14.1). This ensures that the hard palate is horizontal and appears as a single line on the final image. If Frankfort plane is not horizontal and the error is large, the image of the palate can be shown cutting through the apices of the upper teeth. Large errors in positioning Frankfort plane could also result in the upper and lower apices not remaining within the focal trough (Figure 14.1).
- The patient is looking directly ahead (neither turned to the left or right). If the patient is rotated to the left or right, it takes one side of the mandible and maxilla further from

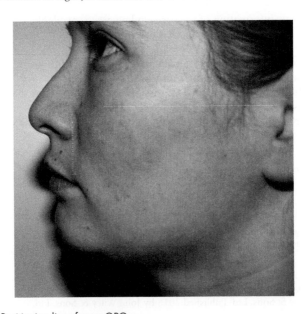

Figure 14.1 Positioning lines for an OPG

ORTHOPANTOMOGRAPHY

the film than the other side. This will result in the magnification of the side that is further from the film, and diagnosis is made more difficult, if not impossible, by the differential magnification of the left and right.

- Get the patient to push out their chest and pull the shoulders back to ensure the neck is straight. If the patient is allowed to slump and the neck curves normally, it can fall within the imaging plane and shows a dense white shadow masking detail of the anterior teeth.
- Set the focal trough to the upper 2/3 interproximal space or to the upper 3 depending on the machine instructions. This places the anterior teeth within the sharp imaging plane (Figure 14.1).
- The patient's tongue should be in the roof of their mouth. This is very difficult to achieve because you cannot see where the tongue is, and if you ask the patient to put their tongue in a particular place, they seem to find it difficult to understand and comply with what you say. If you ask the patient to put their tongue into the roof of their mouth, very often they will raise the tip, but the rest of the tongue tends to fall away from the required position.

There are many different OPG machines in use, and the degree of assistance in obtaining the required ideal position can vary considerably.

Some machines have guide lights for Frankfort plane, median sagittal plane and focal trough, others will have none of these, and older machines may have pull down plastic guides with lines imprinted to help line up the essential markers.

When setting the focal trough, some machines will move the chin rest and therefore the patient into or out of the machine; in others the pivot point itself is moved in or out; and with others there is no manual adjustment of the focal trough.

It is not possible to show all of these and to give detailed instructions within this text.

It is very important that before operating any X-ray equipment you must receive instruction in all aspects of its use from someone who is competent and fully understands the unit.

- The horizontal white line in Figure 14.1 shows the position of Frankfort plane and the vertical white line the position for the focal trough.

All of the positioning requirements are in place to ensure that the image produces the maximum diagnostic information with accuracy.

Any deviation from the optimum position may have an adverse effect on the diagnostic information presented and therefore the accuracy of treatment planning.

Just as we did with the intra-oral image, an accurate assessment of all of the positioning parameters must be made before any diagnosis is attempted.

Again as with intra-oral images, always following the same pattern of assessment will ensure that none of the features are neglected.

OPG IMAGE ASSESSMENT

Area

With any radiograph the first thing to check would be the following:

- Has the whole of the area under examination been included on the image? The required parameters are as follows:

- The condyles of the temporomandibular joints, the angles of the mandible and the symphysis menti (point of the chin).

  This area is a little larger than would necessarily be required for a most diagnostic purposes, but it does give fixed anatomical points of reference.
- On many modern machines the area of exposure can be reduced for children to reduce the radiation dose delivered.

An important point to be kept in mind is that if the larger area is exposed, all of the anatomy visible must be included on the report if the exposure is to be justified under IR(ME)R.

Projection

In this section checks will be made on all of the positional parameters that were used to set up the patient for the OPG.

FRANKFORT PLANE ASSESSMENT

Was Frankfort plane placed in the correct (horizontal) position?

To assess this, look at the white line produced by the borders of the hard palate. Are the anterior and posterior borders superimposed so that they form a single white line? (Figure 14.2a)

If the head is tipped forwards or backwards, the anterior and posterior borders of the palate will move in relation to each other, one will be above the other, and a double rather than a single line will be seen (Figure 14.2b).

If the two lines have only slight separation, it is not of great importance to the image quality, but when they become widely separated as the head is tipped further then one of the lines representing the palate may be shown overlying the upper apices.

When the error of positioning is sufficient for the palate to overlie the apices, there will be difficulty in assessing the mandible, maxilla and teeth. This is because there will be a change in the positional relationship between these structures and there will be distortion of the anatomical detail.

To judge whether the chin is too far down or too far up, you can look at two different features.

If the occlusal plane looks as if the patient is smiling at you, the chin is too far down.

If it looks as if the patient is frowning, the chin is too far up.

Look at the lines of the hard palate. If the top line is made up of two short curves, the chin is up; if the bottom line is two curves, the chin is down.

- The two figures show the appearance of the hard palate related to the position of Frankfort plane. Figure 14.2a shows the palate when Frankfort plane is correct; the palate is a single sharp line. Figure 14.2b shows the palate clearly as two lines, and in addition the occlusal plane looks smiley; this means the chin is too far down. The occlusal plane cannot be used as the primary assessment of Frankfort plane as its appearance (smile, frown, straight) can depend on the shape of the dental arch, even with Frankfort plane horizontal.

ORTHOPANTOMOGRAPHY

(a)

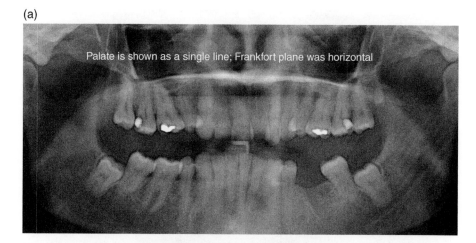

(b)

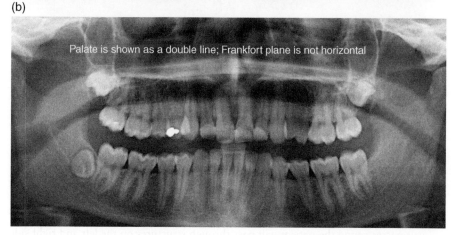

Figure 14.2 (a) Correct hard palate appearance. (b) Incorrect hard palate appearance

- When the palate looks like the one in Figure 14.3, one side a single line and one double, there are a number of potential causes; anatomical variation or positional error, such as; slight tilting or rotation of the head. Where this appearance is seen, a careful check for rotation and tilting is required.

MEDIAN SAGITTAL PLANE ASSESSMENT

Was the median sagittal plane vertical, with the inter pupillary line being horizontally.

There are a number of methods employed for assessing the median sagittal plane, and any conversation with those performing dental radiography will reveal that people adopt and support their own particular favourite.

ORTHOPANTOMOGRAPHY

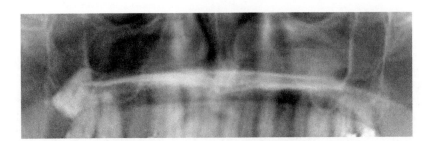

Figure 14.3 Asymmetric hard palate appearance

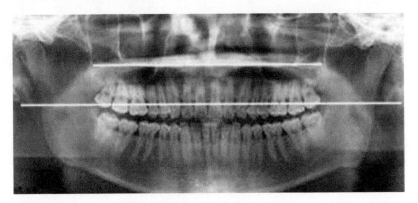

Figure 14.4 Assessment for tilting of the head in OPGs

- The image seen in Figure 14.4 shows the head is not tilted to the left or right as the line joining the left and right extremes of the palate is parallel to the middle of the film.

The reason for checking is that if the head is tilted to the left or right, the X-ray beam as it passes round the patient will pass through structures on the left and right side at differing angles.

This will produce images of the left and right sides that look different because of the distortion.

Not noticing and taking into account the changes in the image caused by tilting the head may lead to errors in the assessment of the patients' condition.

Assessment 1

Check that the top of the condyles of the left and right temporomandibular joints are equal distances from the top of the film or field of exposure.

Assessment 2

Are the left and right angles of the mandible are of equal distances from the bottom of the film or field of exposure?

Assessment 3

Imagine a line from the extreme left and right edges of the palate (place a ruler or other straight edge across if necessary). Is this line parallel to a line drawn across the middle of the film or edge to edge? If so, there is no tilting (Figure 14.4).

Which one of these is best? It's difficult to say. Each of the methods depends to a greater or lesser extent on the symmetry of the patient's anatomy and the ability of the assessor to select identical points on the left and right to make the assessment.

ORTHOPANTOMOGRAPHY

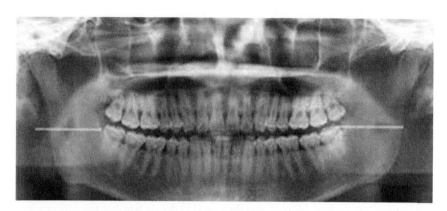

Figure 14.5 Assessing rotation of the head on an OPG

It is probably best to look at all three of the aforementioned, then look at the general bone structure to assess symmetry and then make your value judgement on the position of the median sagittal plane.

Was the patient rotated to the left or right?

Again as with the median sagittal plane and inter-pupillary line, there are a number of methods that can be employed for assessing rotation. They will also depend on the symmetry of the patient's anatomy and the ability of the assessor to select appropriate points of comparison.

Assessment 1

Measure the distance from the angle of the mandible to the symphysis menti. If the distance is equal on both sides, the patient is not rotated; if the distances are different, then there is rotation.

Assessment 2

Measure the full width of the mandibular rami. If the measurement is equal on both sides, the patient is not rotated. If the distances are different, then there is rotation (Figure 14.5).

Assessment 3

Look at the left and right molars. If they look to be of the same size, there is no rotation; if one side looks magnified compared with the other, there is rotation.

Assessment 4

Measure the distance from the interproximal space between the upper central incisors to the bony edge of the ramus on each side. If the measurements are equal, there is no rotation; if they are different, there is some rotation.

Is there a preferred or best option for this assessment? It will once again depend on who you ask but probably the most reliable, but sometimes the most difficult is to assess the relative size of the molars on the left and right.

> • Figure 14.5 shows the measurement of the left and right ramus. The two white lines are of identical length: the one on the left ramus is entirely within the ramus, and the another one on the right extends beyond it. The ramus on the left side is therefore magnified compared with the right. The last molar on the left also looks larger, and the palate although a single line on the left looks double on the right. These asymmetrical appearances between left and right are all due to rotation of the head.

FOCAL TROUGH ASSESSMENT

Was the focal trough set correctly on the interproximal upper 2/3 (or upper 3)?

This is more straightforward than the previous two assessments: look at the anterior teeth, upper and lower 1, 2 and 3.

Are these teeth in focus and the edges appearing sharp on the image? If the answer is yes, then the focal trough was set correctly.

Is it really that simple? No, it isn't. Having looked at 1–3 you also need to look at the rest of the image to make sure the blurring that you see is not due to movement of the patient during the exposure.

Also remember that due to the tomographic effect, an OPG image will never look as sharply in focus as a periapical image.

If the anterior teeth look blurred, you then need to decide whether the patient was too far out of the machine (focal trough to far forward) or was the patient too far into the machine (focal trough too far back).

If the patient is too far out, they will have moved away from the film or sensor; this has the effect of magnifying the image and the teeth then look broad and spade-like.

If the patient is too far forward in the machine (closer to the film or sensor), the teeth will appear very narrow.

Remember with these last two points to take into account what the patients' teeth actually look like, they may be either broad or very narrow. If the teeth look either broad or narrow but are well defined with no blurring, the focal trough is correctly set and the appearance is anatomical.

> • The image here (Figure 14.6) shows the anterior teeth both upper and lower with good fine detail within the limits of an OPG. This indicates that the focal trough was set correctly and there was no movement of the patient during the exposure.

What conclusion can you make if when assessing the focal trough you think that the crowns and incisal edges look sharp and in focus but the apices of the teeth look blurred and indistinct?

When you see this effect, you will probably already have noted that Frankfort plane was not horizontal. The effect occurs because the incisal edges of the teeth biting edge to edge in the groove of the bite block will remain in the focal trough (if it is set correctly) as the head tips forwards or backwards. The apices however (if the head is tipped far enough) will eventually be moved out of the focal trough and will look blurred.

If the head tips chin down, the upper apices effectively move forward and the lower backwards and vice versa.

> • In the diagrams shown in Figure 14.7, the two vertical lines show the area of the focal trough (sharp imaging plane). When Frankfort plane is horizontal, the front teeth are completely within the focal trough. With the head tilted backwards, the upper apices come out of the focal trough when tilted forward the lower apices are outside the required area (Figure 14.7). The features remaining in or being taken out of the focal trough will depend on individual anatomical variations and will only occur in machines with a narrow focal trough.

ORTHOPANTOMOGRAPHY

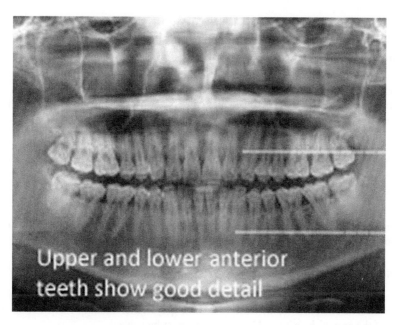

Figure 14.6 OPG assessment of the focal trough

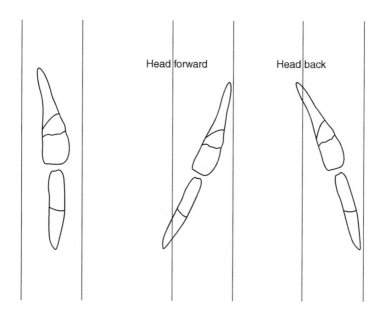

Figure 14.7 Frankfort plane and the focal trough

Was the spine straightened?

  If the spine is allowed to curve naturally, it will be moved closer to the anterior portion of the imaging plane and a partial image of it will appear overlying the anterior teeth.

When this occurs, there will be a white shadow over the teeth, upper and lower 1–3; this will hide the detail completely or make the teeth appear very blurred.

Was the tongue in the roof of the mouth?

If the tongue was not in the roof of the mouth, air lying above it and below the palate will show as a dark shadow. The shadow is rarely dark enough to directly affect the view of structures that the air lies over, but it can be a distraction to the person making the diagnostic assessment.

> • The white line on Figure 14.8 shows the high-density air shadow between the bottom of the palate and top of the tongue.

This completes the part of the assessment that we called the projection, and the remainder follows the same pattern as that for intra-oral radiographs:

Density

Just we did with the periapicals and bitewings, we look first at the directly exposed areas.

Are these areas black or at least very dark grey? After making this assessment the whole of the area to be assessed for diagnosis must be viewed.

Is there sufficient density in all areas to make the required diagnostic assessment?

Contrast

Again assessment is similar to that discussed for periapical and bitewing images. Look at the difference in density between adjacent areas: Do the pulp, dentine and enamel show clearly? Is the density difference between them, wide (good contrast), narrow (poor contrast) or somewhere in between?

When making this assessment it is important that you remember that the contrast shown on an OPG will never be as good as it can be on an intra-oral image. This is because the blurred image of structures not lying in the imaging plane will overlie some of the detail that is of diagnostic interest.

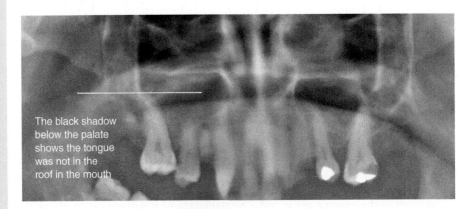

The black shadow below the palate shows the tongue was not in the roof in the mouth

Figure 14.8 OPG, tongue not in the roof of the mouth

ORTHOPANTOMOGRAPHY

Sharpness

This is defined by the level of fine detail that can be seen in the image, and it is something that can only be accurately assessed with some experience.

Experience is needed because the OPG will not produce an image with very well-defined fine structures due to the simultaneous movement of the X-ray tube and the film/sensor during the exposure.

Artefacts

As with intra-oral radiographs the artefacts are features seen on the image that are not part of the patients' anatomy and therefore should not be seen.

Two of the most common are necklaces and earrings.

Earrings will show an actual image on each of the ears and two further shadows higher up near the palate and on each side of the midline.

The one on the right will be the left earring and that on the left is the right earring. They show in this way because of the slight upward angle of the beam on most OPG machines and the direction of the beam as it passes through the earrings.

Necklaces always seem to come to a sharp point at the back of the neck (like the narrow end of an egg). The appearance is caused by the angle of the X-ray beam as it passes round the patient. Because it looks too narrow to be around a neck, it is often not recognised for what it is.

There will also be the usual assessment of image artefacts: scratches, crimp marks, gelatine, sensor marks, etc.

Following this full assessment, the image should be graded on the 1–3 system, and all of the aforementioned must be correct for the film to be graded at 1.

Chapter 15

Other dental radiographic techniques

BISECTING ANGLE PERIAPICAL RADIOGRAPHS

While the paralleling technique is undoubtedly the best and the preferred method for producing periapical and bitewing radiographs, there may be circumstances where it cannot be utilised.

Such circumstances would be:

Recent trauma.
Recent surgery.
Anatomical anomalies.
Shallow palate (there is no room for the film to stand parallel to the teeth).
Narrow arch (no room for a film to sit between the left and right sides of the arch).
Patients with a pronounced gag reflex may be difficult, but in many cases the use of distraction techniques can make a big difference. Examples would be making small circles with a foot or touching each finger to the thumb in turn.
The patient tapping their finger on their chin just above the symphysis menti can also be very effective, as can making the film slightly damp before insertion.

If it does prove impossible to place the film holder or if circumstances dictate that it is not sensible to try, an alternative must be found.

The alternative technique would be the bisecting angle technique. It provides a useful backup where paralleling techniques cannot be used, but the images are not sufficiently accurate for it to be the technique of first choice.

The bisecting angle technique is one of compromise as a number of the requirements specified for perfect imaging geometry are not met:

The film is not parallel to the object.
The central ray is not perpendicular to the film.
The central ray is not perpendicular to the object (tooth).

There will always be some distortion of the image when bisecting angle is employed, and it is the task of the operator to ensure that this distortion is minimised. The bisecting angle method is a compromise trying to ensure that the central ray is not too far from perpendicular in relation to the film and the tooth.

Basic Guide to Dental Radiography, First Edition. Tim Reynolds.
© 2016 John Wiley & Sons, Ltd. Published 2016 by John Wiley & Sons, Ltd.

When the perfect compromise is achieved, there will be distortion of the image but it will have been reduced as far as possible within the limits of this technique.

Positioning the film

The general rules for positioning the film remain the same as those explained for the paralleling technique.

The central (long axis for anterior teeth) (central short axis for posterior teeth) is positioned so that it is coincident (lined up perfectly) with the tooth being investigated or with the appropriate interproximal space.

Then the lower border (upper teeth) or upper border (lower teeth) is positioned 3 mm from the incisal edge or occlusal surface. As with the paralleling technique the gap between the bite surfaces is not important, but placing the film in this position will allow 4 mm of apical tissues to be included.

Unlike the paralleling technique the film is placed in close contact with the tooth or teeth being investigated, but it will not be parallel to the tooth as the bony structures of the maxilla or mandible and the gums will keep the film some distance from the roots.

> • Figure 15.1 shows the relative position between the film and the tooth for the bisecting angle technique. This, none ideal, position cannot be improved because of the anatomy. The angle existing between the film and the tooth becomes greater as we move towards examinations of the anterior teeth. So for anterior teeth the relative position of the film and tooth becomes further from the ideal parallel relationship and distortion increases.

It is also important that the film is supported by a pair of forceps or a specially designed bisecting angle film holder and not by the patients' finger. The reason for this is not related to radiation safety but to imaging geometry. Pushing the film against the teeth with a finger will bend the film and increase the severity of any distortion in the image.

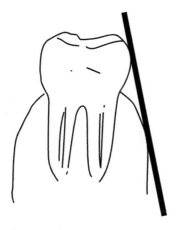

Figure 15.1 Relative film/tooth position for bisecting angle technique

The central ray in bisecting angle

To line up the central ray so that it is perpendicular to either the tooth or the film would create the maximum distortion in the final image.

- Figure 15.2 shows two potential incorrect positions for the central ray for a bisecting angle technique: A is perpendicular to the long axis of the tooth and B is perpendicular to the film. Either of these would produce an unacceptable level of distortion.

To position the central ray correctly, the angle that naturally exists between the film and the tooth must be bisected (halved). This is not easy as with the tooth all that can be seen is the crown and much of the film is pushed up behind the gum so the angle between the tooth and the film is being assessed with a very limited view of either of them.

- Figure 15.3 shows the correct position of the central ray, B, perpendicular to the line, A, bisecting the angle between the tooth and the film. Drawing this technique accurately to scale on a piece of paper using a protractor and ruler gives an 8–15% increase in root length, depending on which teeth are being examined. This is not too critical if you remember to apply it to any measurements. However any error in assessing the bisecting angle and directing the central ray, even small errors, will make big changes to the elongation or foreshortening of the image. The problem is that although you can see the image is elongated or foreshortened, you do not know by how much accurate measurements cannot therefore be taken.

The difficulty in making an accurate assessment of the bisecting angle means that many people rely on the general guidelines that can be found in many general or specific dental radiographic texts. These guidelines give an approximate central ray angle for each area of the mouth.

The guide is sufficient to give a reasonable result in the majority of cases, but it must always be remembered that where there is an unusual bite, the angle between the tooth and the film will not conform to the average. In such a case independent assessment of the angles will be necessary to avoid excessive elongation or foreshortening.

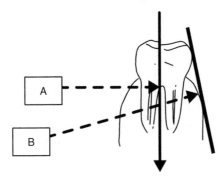

Figure 15.2 Incorrect central ray positioning in bisecting angle techniques

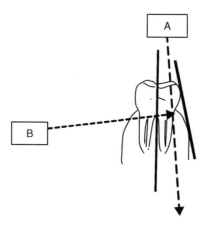

Figure 15.3 Correct central ray position for bisecting angle

Bisecting angle guide to central ray positioning

876	54	3	21	Upper arch
↓	↓	↓	↓	
20–25°	30–35°	45–50°	50–55°	

0–5°	5–10°	15–20°	20°	
↑	↑	↑	↑	
876	54	3	21	Lower arch

For the upper arch the angles refer to start with the central ray horizontal and then angle downwards, and for the lower arch start with the central ray horizontal and angle upwards (Figure 15.4).

NB: If it is necessary to perform a bisecting angle technique, remember that the angles given are a general guide only and the actual angle used must depend on the assessment of the position of the tooth, the film and the imaginary line bisecting the angle between them. For the upper arch the position of the upper positioning line (Chapter 13) and for the lower arch the position of the lower positioning line (Chapter 13) must also be taken into account.

Assessment of the bisecting angle image

There is no need at this time to write in detail about the assessment of a bisecting angle periapical radiograph.

The reason for making this statement is that the method used for the assessment follows closely that used for the paralleling technique.

The same general headings will be used: area, projection, density, contrast, sharpness, artefacts and grade.

The one difference will be in the assessment of the vertical (caudo-cranial) angle.

When assessing this angle for paralleling techniques, two methods were used:

1. For molar teeth we checked that the crowns were in profile and that opposing cusps were not shown (effectively looking into the occlusal surface). This assessment is shown in Figure 13.21a and b.

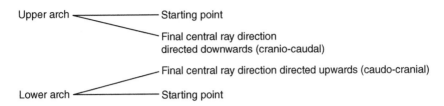

Figure 15.4 Central ray directions for bisecting angle techniques

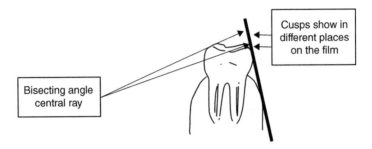

Figure 15.5 Demonstration of molar cusps in bisecting angle technique

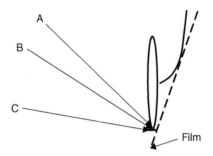

Figure 15.6 Incisal edge position in bisecting angle technique

An assessment of this type will not work for bisecting angle techniques because the central ray will never be passing directly across the top of the crown but will in a position that always projects buccal cusps onto a different part of the film to the palatal or lingual (Figure 15.5).

2. For incisors the assessment of the vertical angle was made by measuring the distance from the incisal edge to the edge of the film. If the paralleling technique is correctly performed, there is a 3 mm gap from the tooth to the edge of the film. If the vertical angle is wrong, the gap is either reduced or increased (Figure 13.22b). This reduction or increase in the gap occurs because there is a significant distance between the tooth and the film.

With the bisecting angle the edge of the tooth is in contact with the film so changing the vertical angle will not change the position of the image of the incisal edge on the film (Figure 15.6).

- Three very different central ray angles (A, B and C) all show the incisal edge of the tooth in the same place in relation to the edge of the film. So the position of the incisal edge cannot be used to assess the vertical angle (Figure 15.6).

Although the methods described in Chapter 13 for checking the vertical angle are not appropriate for the bisecting angle, the method used (elongation and foreshortening) will be familiar to most people. It is in fact often quoted in error for assessment of paralleling technique periapical radiographs (remember that elongation and foreshortening do not occur if the film is maintained in a position parallel to the tooth).

Incorrect direction of the central ray in bisecting angle techniques will produce elongation or foreshortening of the image. The part of the image that is most affected will be the root length, because it is the root that is at some distance from the film in this technique.

- Figure 15.7 shows the bisecting line (X) and three potential positions for the central ray: (A) shows the correct angle and the position of the image of the apex on the film, (B) shows a shallow angle with the apex being stretched down the film (elongation), and (C) shows a steep angle pushing the apex further up the film giving foreshortening.

For a general rule to remember what sort of error in central ray positioning will produce elongation or foreshortening, you need only to think of being out in the sun.

Early in the morning or in the evening when the sun is low in the sky (at a shallow angle), the shadows cast will be long.

At midday with the sun high overhead (steep angle), the shadows cast will be short.

The level of foreshortening or elongation produced by an incorrect angle of the central ray for the bisecting angle technique will be much greater for anterior teeth than for posterior teeth.

The reason for the different levels of elongation or foreshortening is the much greater angle between the tooth and the film when taking radiographs of the anterior teeth.

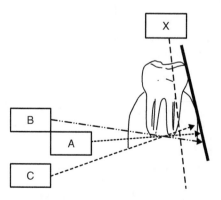

Figure 15.7 Elongation and foreshortening in bisecting angle techniques

OCCLUSAL RADIOGRAPHS

Prior to the introduction of the orthopantomogram X-ray machines, full mouth orthodontic surveys were carried out through occlusal techniques. The film used for this technique was, although much larger, very similar in construction to standard dental X-ray film.

In order to produce a full examination of the teeth, maxilla and body of the mandible, five exposures were required. Two different projections were required for the mandible and three for the maxilla.

For the maxilla, one occlusal film would be placed centrally in the mouth so that the long central axis of the film was lined up with the median sagittal plane and the other two films were slightly offset from the centre to provide images of the left and right sides.

> • Figure 15.8 shows the positioning of three occlusal films to provide complete images of the maxillary arch. The dashed lines indicate a tangent to the curve of the arch (line that just touches the edge of the curve), and the arrows show the general direction of the central ray of the X-ray beam. The central ray hits the tangent of the curve at an angle of 90°. This particular technique for investigating the maxilla is now rarely employed. The most likely, though still uncommon, image you will see is that produced by the film in the centre of the arch: an upper standard occlusal radiograph.

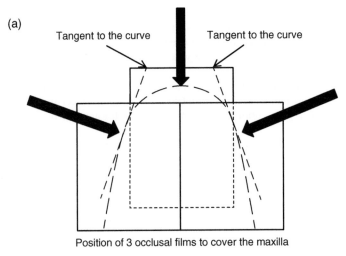

(a)

Tangent to the curve   Tangent to the curve

Position of 3 occlusal films to cover the maxilla

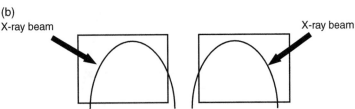

(b)
X-ray beam   X-ray beam

Figure 15.8 (a) Occlusal film positions for full cover of the maxillary arch. (b) Alternative film position for oblique images

OTHER DENTAL RADIOGRAPHIC

The films for the left and right oblique views are displaced to the side being imaged. An alternative to this is to place the film so that it is positioned transversely in the middle of the mouth with the central ray being directed as already shown.

The technique used is a matter of personal choice with either one performed correctly producing a perfectly good image and each causing a similar level of discomfort for the patient. Whichever method you use the film has to be in a position to include the teeth and maxilla of the side being imaged so there will be similar disruption of the patients' lips and cheek. The central anterior film is still required.

> • Figure 15.8b shows the alternative film position for oblique occlusals. The disadvantage is that you cannot show so much of the posterior parts of the maxilla.

In addition to the central ray hitting the tangent of the curve at 90°, it should also hit the middle of the film at the correct vertical angle for minimising the distortion of the image.

There will be distortion because as with periapical bisecting angle techniques the film is not parallel to the teeth. There is in fact a much greater angle between the teeth and the film than is the case with periapicals. This large angle of separation between the teeth and the film has the potential to produce much more severe elongation or foreshortening than is the case with periapical radiography.

Although occlusal radiography is a bisecting angle technique, the angle between the teeth and the film is:

1. Difficult to assess
2. Variable because the film covers a larger area of the arch

The two aforementioned factors mean that rather than trying to make an assessment of the angle between the teeth and the film then bisecting it, the use of the guideline angles of approximately 60–65° for the anterior projection and 50–55° for the oblique ones will produce good results in the majority of cases. It is only in cases of extreme malocclusion that modifications will be required.

Standard positioning for the upper central occlusal image

The patient is seated erect with the median sagittal plane vertical and the upper positioning line horizontal.

The film is placed with its long axis coincident with the median sagittal plane and with approximately 1.5 cm of film protruding from the mouth.

The central ray is angled downwards approximately 60° and centred so that it passes just below the nasion and through the centre of the hard palate.

> • Figure 15.9 shows the typical beam alignment for an upper occlusal radiography. Note the angle of the cone and the fact that the central line of the cone (and therefore the central ray of the beam) passes just below the nasion, above the upper apices and through the centre of the hard palate.

OTHER DENTAL RADIOGRAPHIC

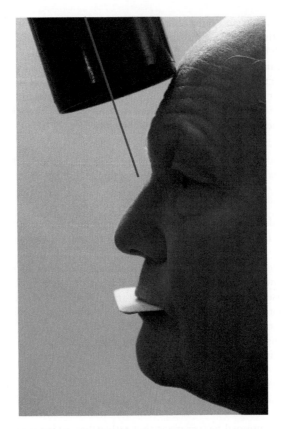

Figure 15.9 Beam alignment for upper occlusal radiography

- Figure 15.10 shows the typical appearance of an upper central occlusal radiograph. Errors in the vertical angle will cause large-scale elongation or foreshortening of the teeth and distortion of the image of the palate. It is very important that the image quality and potential distortion are assessed prior to any diagnostic conclusions being drawn.

Upper oblique occlusal imaging

- The photographs shown in Figure 15.11 give the positioning of the film and cone for the left and right upper oblique occlusal projections. No further detail or discussion will be dedicated to this technique as it is highly unlikely that you will see it other than in archived interesting cases or in radiographic texts. In fact all occlusal techniques are rare in dental radiography today as there are much more effective imaging techniques for the maxilla.

OTHER DENTAL RADIOGRAPHIC

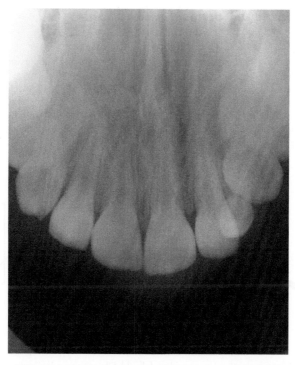

Figure 15.10 The general appearance of an upper standard occlusal radiograph. Though it is usual to see approximately 1 to 1.5 cm of unexposed film anteriorly with a slightly elliptical shape to the unexposed area, errors in the vertical angle will cause large-scale elongation or foreshortening of the teeth and distortion of the image of the palate. It is very important that the image quality and potential distortion are assessed prior to any diagnostic conclusions being drawn. Source: Reproduced with permission of Katrina Hickenbotham

(a)   (b)

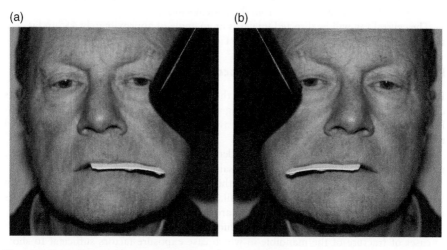

Figure 15.11 Upper oblique occlusal X-ray tube positioning

OTHER DENTAL RADIOGRAPHIC

Positioning for lower occlusal radiographs

- Figure 15.12a shows two occlusal films in place for the lower (mandibular) arch; these films together with the three shown in the upper (maxillary) arch in Figure 15.8a would have been used to complete a full orthodontic survey prior to the introduction of OPG machines and techniques. The arrows indicate the general direction of the central ray of the X-ray beam. In modern dentistry this technique will not be seen and the film position shown in Figure 15.12b, lower central occlusal, is the technique most likely to be seen though all occlusal radiography is rare.

(a)   (b)

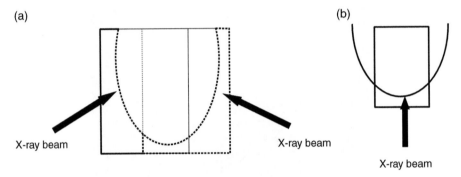

X-ray beam   X-ray beam

X-ray beam

Figure 15.12 (a) Film positions to complete full. (b) Film position for imaging of the standard lower occlusal

The lower central occlusal image is designed to demonstrate the lower anterior teeth and the area of the symphysis menti.

The patient will be seated with the median sagittal plane vertical and the lower positioning line (described on page 130) horizontal.

The film is placed with its long axis coincident with the median sagittal plane and with approximately 1.5 cm protruding from the patient's mouth.

The central ray will be directed upwards at an angle of approximately 45° and is centred directly through the symphysis menti (Figure 15.13a and b).

Positioning for infero-superior occlusal imaging

Infero-superior refers to the direction of the central ray as with other terms such as cranio-caudal; it is a descriptive term stating where the beam starts and where it is travelling to. An infero-superior central ray is travelling generally from the bottom (inferior) towards the top (superior).

The technique is primarily designed to demonstrate the soft tissues of the floor of the mouth when investigating submandibular salivary glands and their ducts for stones.

To show stones in the glands and ducts, the exposure factors must be much lower than would be necessary to show the bony detail. If the exposure is too high, the soft tissues and stones may be penetrated so that they are not demonstrated on the image.

The technique has also been used to demonstrate the position of displaced fragments in cases of fracture of the mandible in which case exposure factors sufficient to show bony detail would be utilised.

(a)   (b)

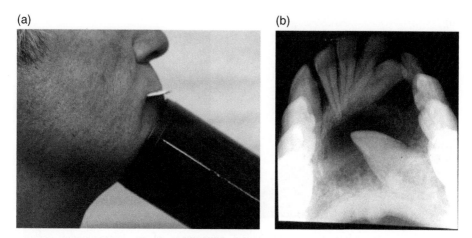

Figure 15.13 (a) Lower occlusal positioning. (b) Typical appearance of a lower central occlusal radiograph. Source: Reproduced with permission of Katrina Hickenbotham

Technique

The film is inserted, tube side downwards with the central axis coincident with the median sagittal plane in exactly the same position as it was for the lower central occlusal (Figure 15.12b).

The head will be tipped backwards so that the X-ray tube can be positioned directly below the mandible and the central ray directed perpendicular to the film.

The central ray should be positioned to pass approximately 2.5 cm behind the symphysis menti and on along the median sagittal plane.

- Figure 15.14a shows the standard positioning for an infero-superior occlusal projection. The white line represents the position of the central ray entering 2.5 cm below the symphysis menti and hitting the centre of the film at 90°.
- Figure 15.14b shows the typical appearance of infero-superior occlusal radiograph; note that the whole of the floor of the mouth is seen along with a plan view of the mandible. Little information regarding the teeth will be evident unless there are extreme malpositions that bring them out of the line of the mandible.

CEPHALOMETRIC IMAGING

Cephalic or cephalad refers to the head and metric to measurement; therefore cephalometric imaging is about measurement of the head or features related to it.

The examination (lateral cephalometry) is used in orthodontics to assess malocclusions and disproportions in the cranial and facial profiles.

For full assessments the image must be as accurate as possible and free of positioning errors that could produce false appearances and/or measurements.

It is also important that the bony and soft tissues are demonstrated on a single image. This could be achieved with very high kilovoltages to reduce contrast but modern equipment designed for cephalometry; a wedge filter is incorporated in the design.

OTHER DENTAL RADIOGRAPHIC

(a)   (b)

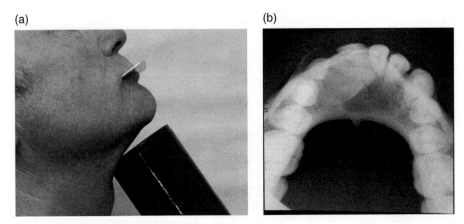

The thicker end of the wedge is positioned over the facial area to absorb some of the beam and to reduce the intensity of X-rays passing through the facial area to expose the film or sensor. The bony areas are exposed to the full beam and are therefore more heavily exposed. In this way all of the tissues can be demonstrated on the image.

Positioning the patient for cephalometry

The patient should be standing erect with their median sagittal plane parallel to the film/sensor and the inter-pupillary line (a line drawn directly between the pupils of the two eyes) perpendicular to the film/sensor (The Inter-pupillary line is horizontal).

These two positioning parameters ensure that there is no tilting or rotation of the head. There should be molar occlusion and Frankfort plane should be horizontal.

Frankfort plane is placed horizontally to ensure that the posterior borders of the body and rami of the mandible are projected clear of the cervical spine.

Central ray

The central ray of the X-ray beam should be perpendicular to the film/sensor and should be directed to a point 2.5 cm behind the outer canthus of the eye (the canthus is the joining point of the upper and lower eye lids.

- Figure 15.15 shows the two major positioning planes for lateral cephalometry: A shows the median sagittal plane that is positioned parallel to the film/sensor and B shows the inter-pupillary line that is positioned perpendicular to the film/sensor.

Assessment of the cephalometric image

As with previous imaging techniques described, the cephalometric image should be assessed to a particular pattern to ensure that the assessment is as full as it can be.

The pattern will follow that previously used, utilising the following titles: area, projection, density, contrast, sharpness and artefacts.

OTHER DENTAL RADIOGRAPHIC

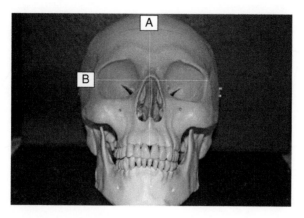

Figure 15.15 Positioning lines for cephalometry

Lateral cephalometry image assessment

Area

Does the film include the frontal bone, the graduated metal measure over the nasion, the symphysis menti, the bodies of the cervical vertebrae and the soft tissues over the face and neck?
Is the graduated marker in contact with the nasion adequately demonstrated? This must be shown as it is an indicator of the amount of magnification of midline structures in the patient, the markers on it must be visible.

Projection

Was Frankfort plane horizontal? This is assessed by looking at two features:
Is the hard palate horizontal and are the posterior borders of the mandibular rami shown clear of the anterior border of the cervical vertebrae?
Was there any rotation of the head?
In the centre of the skull, there is a feature called the sella turcica where the pituitary gland sits in the middle part of it (the pituitary fossa). At the back of the sella, there are two bony projections, one on each side, called the posterior clinoid processes.

If the head is rotated, both of these processes can be seen one in front of the other.

- Figure 15.16a shows the posterior clinoid processes superimposed. It looks as if there is only one, not two. This is the appearance when there is no rotation of the head.
- Figure 15.16b shows both clinoid processes one in front of the other; this is the appearance of the processes when there is rotation of the head.

Was there any tilting of the head?
This can again be assessed by looking at the posterior clinoid processes but it can also be the floor of the pituitary fossa that gives the answer (Figure 15.17).

Was the image produced with molar occlusion? This feature requires no explanation as it is easily assessed.

OTHER DENTAL RADIOGRAPHIC

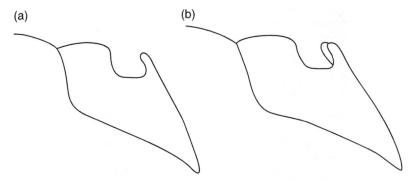

Figure 15.16 (a) Superimposed clinoid. (b) Clinoid processes not superimposed

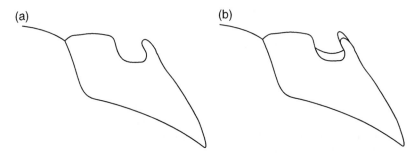

Figure 15.17 (a) No tilting of the head. (b) Appearance with the head tilted

- Figure 15.17a shows both the floor of the pituitary fossa and the posterior clinoid processes as single items meaning that there is no tilting of the head.
- Figure 15.17b shows two lines to the floor of the fossa and both clinoid processes in both cases the features are demonstrated one above the other indicating that the head was tilted either to the left or the right.

Density
Two assessments are made of the density:

1. Are the directly exposed areas black or dark grey?
2. Is there sufficient density to clearly identify all of the necessary bony features?

Contrast
Is the contrast sufficient to identify not only the necessary bony landmarks but also the soft tissues of the face and neck?

Sharpness
Is there sufficient demonstration of the fine detail to allow the accurate assessment of the measurements and the general condition of the bony structures?
The sharpness of a radiograph will usually be perfectly adequate, and it is only if the patient has moved that there will be a problem.

OTHER DENTAL RADIOGRAPHIC

RARELY USED TECHNIQUES

Here we will mention but not discuss in detail some techniques that are rarely, if ever, used in modern dentistry though some specialised centres may use them occasionally.

Parallax projections

Parallax projections are designed to demonstrate the relative positions of structures or to identify and assess individual roots or root canals for molar teeth.

In general radiography if it is necessary to identify the precise position of a structure, the patient can be turned through 90° to perform what is called a lateral (from the side) projection.

Simply taking a radiograph from a single direction cannot give all of the required information. We may be able to say one structure or feature is higher than the other and more to the right, but we would not know which one was further forward. Producing a second radiograph from the side would give this information.

> • Figure 15.18a (the postero-anterior chest X-ray) shows a shadow in the right close to the heart border, but we do not know if it is actually close to the border of the heart towards the front of the chest or is it at the back of the lung field. The second (lateral) radiography clearly gives the information we require; the lesion is at the back.

When considering dental radiography it is clear that it will not be possible to take a second radiograph at 90° to the original; this is what the parallax projection is for.

> • Figure 15.19a shows the result of a standard radiograph. The roots of the tooth in question are superimposed and clear visualisation is not possible. Figure 15.19b shows the effect of parallax techniques where the X-ray beam is directed across the tooth. This oblique imaging separates the roots so that each can be individually visualised.

(a)   (b)

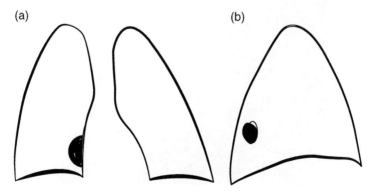

Figure 15.18 (a) Postero-anterior chest. (b) Lateral chest

OTHER DENTAL RADIOGRAPHIC

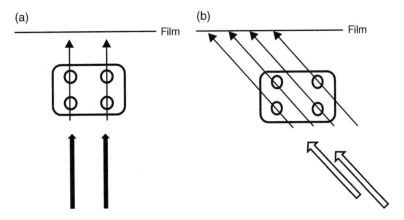

Figure 15.19 (a) Standard radiographic image. (b) Parallax imaging techniques

Lateral oblique mandible (dissociated laterals)

The technique (lateral oblique mandible) was designed to give a radiographic image of the left and right sides of the body of the mandible with two exposures. It would provide information on trauma and pathology of the bony mandible and of the premolars and molars.

Using an OPG or similar-sized cassette, both projections could be produced on a single film. Although it could usefully provide information, this technique is so rare as to be considered to have fallen out of the repertoire of dental radiography. In fact it is highly unlikely that you would see the technique performed even in large hospital X-ray departments.

To perform the examination, the head is first tilted over towards the side to be examined (this is to separate the two sides of the mandible) and the head is then rotated

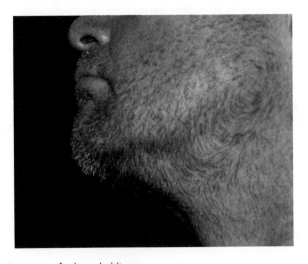

Figure 15.20 Positioning for lateral oblique

forward to bring the body of the mandible into contact with the surface of the cassette (Figure 15.20).

- With the head in this position, a second view of the opposite side (if required) could with careful positioning and centring be produced on the opposite side of the cassette.

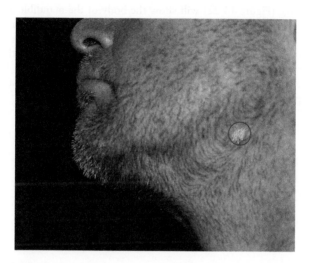

Figure 15.21 The standard centring point 2.5 cm below and in front of the angle of the mandible is shown by the red circle on the jaw. The idea is for the central ray to pass approximately through the body of the mandible in contact with the film cassette

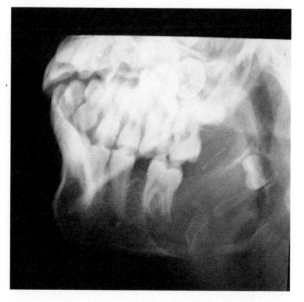

Figure 15.22 Oblique mandible image. Source: Reproduced with permission of katrina Hickenbotham

The body of the mandible now lies in contact with the cassette. The central ray should be directed through a point 2.5 cm below and 2.5 cm in front of the angle of the mandible remote from the cassette and passes through the centre of the body of the mandible in contact with the cassette (Figure 15.21).

Lateral oblique mandible image

The resulting image (Figure 15.22) will show the body of the mandible and the molars, possibly the premolars free of the overlying shadow of the body of the mandible on the opposite side.

Although this text has now included some radiographic techniques that are rare or even obsolete, it will not cover the technique of cone beam CT scanning. This is because it is a highly specialised technique that does not fall within the scope of a basic guide to dental radiography.

Appendix A
Adequate training

Practitioners and operators shall have successfully completed training, including theoretical knowledge and practical experience in:

1. Such of the subjects detailed in section A as are relevant to their functions as practitioner or operator
2. Such of the subjects detailed in section B as are relevant to their specific area of practice

A Radiation production, radiation protection and statutory obligations relating to ionising radiations

1 Fundamental Physics of Radiation

  1.1 Properties of Radiation

    Attenuation of ionising radiation

    Scattering and absorption

  1.2 Radiation Hazards and Dosimetry

    Biological effects of radiation

    Risk/benefits of radiation

    Dose optimisation

    Absorbed dose, dose equivalent, effective dose and their units

  1.3 Special Attention Areas

    Pregnancy and potential pregnancy

    Infants and children

    Medical and biomedical research

    Health screening

    High-dose techniques

2 Management and Radiation Protection of the Patient

  2.1 Patient Selection

    Justification of the individual exposure

    Patient identification and consent

    Use of existing appropriate radiological information

    Alternative techniques

    Clinical Evaluation of outcomes for Medico-legal issues

Basic Guide to Dental Radiography, First Edition. Tim Reynolds.
© 2016 John Wiley & Sons, Ltd. Published 2016 by John Wiley & Sons, Ltd.

2.2 Radiation Protection
General radiation protection
Use of radiation protection devices
Patient
Personal
Procedures for untoward incidents involving overexposure to ionising radiation
3 Statutory Requirements and Advisory Aspects
3.1 Statutory Requirements
Regulations
Local rules and procedures
Individual responsibilities relating to medical exposures
Responsibility for radiation safety
Routine inspection and testing of equipment
Notification of faults and health department hazard warnings
Clinical audit

B Diagnostic radiology, radiotherapy and nuclear medicine
4 Diagnostic Radiology
4.1 General
Fundamentals of radiological anatomy
Fundamentals of radiological techniques
Production of X-rays
Equipment selection and use
Factors affecting radiation dose
Dosimetry
Quality assurance and quality control
4.2 Specialised Techniques
Image intensification/fluoroscopy
Digital fluoroscopy
Computed tomography scanning
Interventional procedures
Vascular imaging
4.3 Fundamentals of Image Acquisition
Image quality versus. radiation dose
Conventional film processing
Additional image formats, acquisition storage and display

FURTHER READING

Schedule 2, Statutory Instruments 2000 No. 1059, *The Ionising Radiations (Medical Exposures) Regulations 2000*. London: The Stationary Office Limited, 2000.

The remaining parts of the schedule are not relevant to dental radiography.

Remember if you perform any practical task related to dental radiography – processing films/phosphor plates, loading film holders, pressing the exposure button, etc – you must have studied and been tested in sufficient items from this schedule as will qualify as adequate training.

Radiation hazards (radiobiological aspects of exposure), radiation protection, quality control and audit will be necessary no matter how small a part you play in the procedure.

Even the smallest practical task could affect the quality of the image and the dose to the patient. These will have influence on the diagnostic information on the radiography and the safety of the patient, so ensuring your competence through training and assessment is essential.

Schedule 2; Ionising Radiations (Medical Exposures) Regulations 2000 (SI 1059).

Appendix B

Image quality troubleshooting

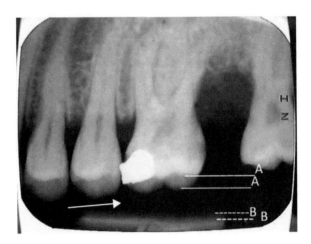

Figure B.1

Figure B.1 demonstrates:

1. Two images of the top edge of the bite block, one very white and one grey and blurred, both marked as B
2. Buccal and palatal cusps separated, both marked as A

- Both of these faults indicate an incorrect cranio-caudal (vertical) angle.
- The reason for this is the patient has not bitten down on the block (large space between bite block and occlusal surface (arrow 1)).
- This has occurred because the film has been placed too close to the teeth and it has caught on the palate, the patient can't close, and the holder and film have tilted from the required position parallel to the teeth.
- **Remember the film should be close to the median sagittal plane.**

Basic Guide to Dental Radiography, First Edition. Tim Reynolds.
© 2016 John Wiley & Sons, Ltd. Published 2016 by John Wiley & Sons, Ltd.

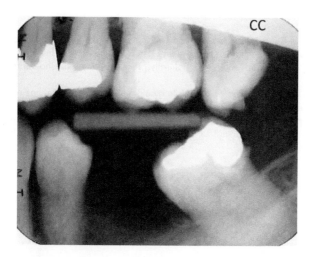

Figure B.2

- The bitewing image shows a fault that is easily identified (Figure B.2).
- The letters C,C indicates a large clear (unexposed) area on the image.
- This is cone cut and is due entirely to the failure to direct the central ray of the beam to the middle of the film.
- It is not due to misdirection of either the caudio-cranial (vertical) or mesio-distal (lateral) angles, though in some cases, those faults may also be present.

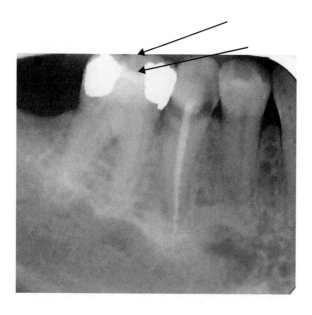

Figure B.3

- Here in Figure B.3 we see the buccal and lingual cusps (marked by the arrows) clearly separated and the bite surface of the teeth close up to the edge of the film rather than there being a 3 mm gap. The gap is naturally produced by the film holder if used properly.
- The bite surface is in contact with the bite block, meaning the patient has bitten properly on the holder.
- The fault separation of cusps and no 3 mm gap is entirely caused by a failure to correctly line up the caudio-cranial (vertical) angle of the central ray with the arm of the holder.

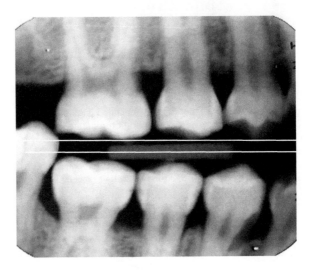

Figure B.4

- The bitewing radiograph, Figure B.4, shows the effect of palatal displacement; the upper teeth are shown to a greater extent than the lower. I have often heard this being attributed to an incorrect caudio-cranial (vertical) angle. It is however invariably due to the film or sensor being placed too close to the teeth. The result is that the film/sensor catches on the lower sulcus and is pushed upwards, or it can catch in the palate and be pushed down to produce lingual displacement. In the example given here, the film has been pushed up out of its correct position in the holder with no other changes to the technique.
- We know the film is pushed out of the holder because the centre line of the film does not lie through the centre line of the bite block (the two white lines should lie on top of each other).
- The caudio-cranial angle is correct; sharp image of the bite block and crowns of the teeth in profile.

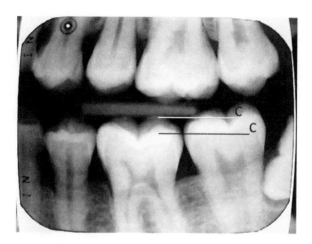

Figure B.5

- Here in Figure B.5 we see lingual displacement, but in this case the caudio-cranial angle is also incorrect. Opposing cusps are indicated by the letters C, C.
- The displacement has not been caused by the caudio-cranial angle. It is again caused by bringing the teeth and film too close together: the film has been pushed out of the holder but the holder has also tilted in the mouth. Following the new line of the holder produces the incorrect caudio-cranial angle.
- There would have been displacement even had the angle been correct.

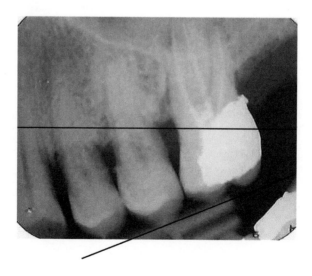

Figure B.6

- Here in Figure B.6 we see again the effect of trying to position the film too close to the teeth.
- The film has contacted the palate and has rotated in the holder (the line through the bite block and the line through the centre of the film should be parallel to each other).
- The holder has also tilted in the patients' mouth so that the film is no longer parallel to the teeth and following the holder produces an incorrect cranio-caudal angle.
- The result is a foreshortened image of the type that should not occur when using a film holder.

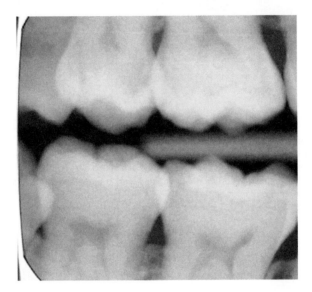

Figure B.7

- Figure B.7 shows the potential effect of the mesio-distal (lateral) angle being incorrectly directed. The sharp white shadows are the areas of overlap between the teeth; the white shadow is caused by the additional attenuation produced by passing the beam through overlapping areas of the teeth.
- The appearance could also be caused by an overcrowded mouth even if the mesio-distal angle were correct.
- The operator would know if there was crowding as they would have seen inside the patients' mouth.

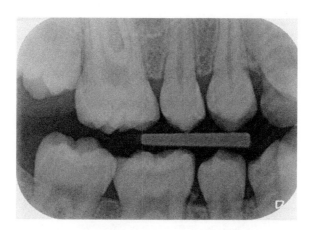

Figure B.8

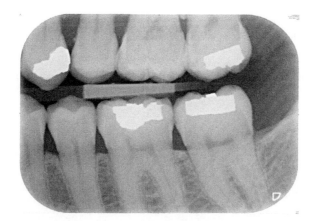

Figure B.9

- Figures B.8 and B.9 show two more examples of displacement; Figure B.8 showing palatal displacement, Figure B.9 lingual.
- In each case it is due to the film being positioned too close to the teeth and the film being pushed out of the holder. (We see the centre of the film is not lined up with the centre of the bite block, its natural position in a bitewing.)
- The holder has not tilted and the central ray remains perpendicular to the centre of the film. We know this because the crowns are in profile (occlusal surface not seen) and the bite block shows as a clear sharp rectangle.

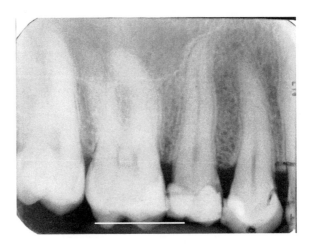

Figure B.10

- Figure B.10 has a white line indicating the level of the top of the bite block. Careful inspection seems to show some molar cusps embedded deep in the block. This cannot be the case as they can only rest in contact with it. The effect is a geometric one caused by a fault in the cranio-caudal (vertical) angle. The angle being incorrect has projected the cusps over the bite block.

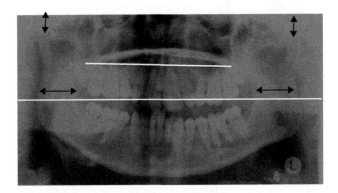

Figure B.11

- Figure B.11, shown previously, demonstrates a number of problems that may be apparent when assessing an OPG. It is often the case that a number of different faults will be seen in a single image.
- The double-headed vertical arrows extending up from the condyles of the TMJ are of equal length but one just touches the top of the image field while the other extends well above it. This means one TMJ is closer to the top of the film than the other (the median sagittal plane is tilted).
- This is confirmed by the two white lines; one joining the lateral parts of the palate and one across the long axis of the film. These two lines should be parallel; the fact that they are not is a confirmation that the median sagittal plane is tilted.
- The two horizontal double-headed arrows are also of equal length, one just fills the width of the ramus, the other falls well short. This indicates that the head is rotated.
- The palate is a single line on one side but double on the other. This means that the Frankfort plane is horizontal; the double line is created by the rotation and tilt (either one by itself could produce this appearance).
- There is also a black shadow immediately below the palate. This means that the tongue was not placed in the roof of the mouth.

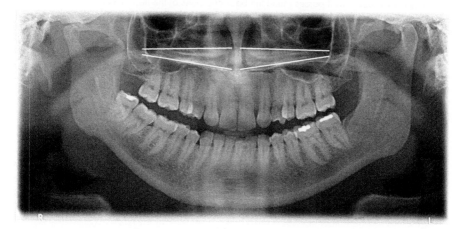

Figure B.12

- Figure B.12 shows clearly that the image of the anterior and posterior portions of the palate are separated and show as two lines on the image: the white lines added, indicate their position. Frankfort plane is not horizontal. Two things tell us that the chin is too far down:

1. The anterior part of the palate is lower than posterior wide (v) shape curving down to the center.
2. The occlusal plane looks like a smile.

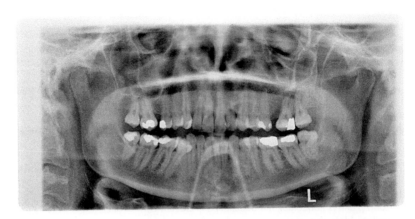

Figure B.13

- The OPG Figure B.13 shows the typical appearance of a necklace artefact. It is often not recognised because of the sharply curved appearance at the back. This is due to the angle of the beam as it passes round the back and sides of the neck. If earrings are left in, four images are seen, one on each ear and a second shadow of each one close to the palates just either side of the midline.

Index

Basic Guide to Dental Radiography, First Edition. Tim Reynolds.
© 2016 John Wiley & Sons, Ltd. Published 2016 by John Wiley & Sons, Ltd.

Printed and bound by CPI Group (UK) Ltd, Croydon, CR0 4YY

12/01/2025

14624493-0001